Until recently, the standardization of diagnosis and assessment of personality disorders has lagged considerably behind that for most other mental disorders. The IPDE is a new instrument which can produce through its two modules diagnoses in accordance with both ICD-10 and DSM-IV criteria. The IPDE is a semistructured clinical interview that provides a means of arriving at the diagnosis of major categories of personality disorders and of assessing personality traits in a standardized and reliable way. It is unique in that it secures reliable information in different cultural settings. Written by leading international authorities, this volume forms an invaluable reference manual to the IPDE instrument. Its first section includes an overview of the results of the worldwide field trials of the interview and discussion of the current status of diagnosis and assessment research. The second section detailing the full interview schedule and scoring system for the instrument will further facilitate its use by both clinician and researcher.

Assessment and diagnosis of personality disorders

Assessment and diagnosis of personality disorders

The ICD-10 international personality disorder examination (IPDE)

Edited by

Armand W. Loranger, Cornell University Medical College,

Aleksandar Janca, World Health Organization,

and

Norman Sartorius, University of Geneva

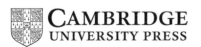

CAMBRIDGE
UNIVERSITY PRESS

PUBLISHED BY THE PRESS SYNDICATE OF THE UNIVERSITY OF CAMBRIDGE
The Pitt Building, Trumpington Street, Cambridge CB2 1RP, United Kingdom

CAMBRIDGE UNIVERSITY PRESS
The Edinburgh Building, Cambridge CB2 2RU, United Kingdom
40 West 20th Street, New York, NY 10011-4211, USA
10 Stamford Road, Oakleigh, Melbourne 3166, Australia

First published 1997

Printed in the United Kingdom at the University Press, Cambridge

Typeset in Times 10pt

A catalogue record for this book is available from the British Library

Library of Congress Cataloguing in Publication data

Assessment and diagnosis of personality disorders: the International Personality Disorder
Examination (IPDE)/edited by Armand W. Loranger, Aleksandar Janca, and Norman
Sartorius.
    p. cm.
Includes index.
ISBN 0-521-58043-9 (hardback)
1. International Personality Disorder Examination.   2. Personality disorders–Diagnosis.
I. Loranger, Armand W. (Armand Walter), 1930– .   II. Janca, A.   III. Sartorius, N.
[DNLM: 1. Personality Disorders – diagnosis.   2. Psychiatric Status Rating Scales.
3. Personality Assessment.   WM 190 A846 1997]
RC544.A87   1997
616.85'8–dc21   96-45992 CIP
DNLM/DLC
for Library of Congress

ISBN 0 521 58043 9 hardback

TAG

Contents

Assessment and diagnosis of personality disorders

The ICD-10 international personality disorder examination (IPDE)

Edited by

Armand W. Loranger, Cornell University Medical College,

Aleksandar Janca, World Health Organization,

and

Norman Sartorius, University of Geneva

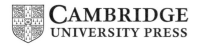

CAMBRIDGE
UNIVERSITY PRESS

PUBLISHED BY THE PRESS SYNDICATE OF THE UNIVERSITY OF CAMBRIDGE
The Pitt Building, Trumpington Street, Cambridge CB2 1RP, United Kingdom

CAMBRIDGE UNIVERSITY PRESS
The Edinburgh Building, Cambridge CB2 2RU, United Kingdom
40 West 20th Street, New York, NY 10011-4211, USA
10 Stamford Road, Oakleigh, Melbourne 3166, Australia

© World Health Organization 1997

First published 1997

Printed in the United Kingdom at the University Press, Cambridge

Typeset in Times 10pt

A catalogue record for this book is available from the British Library

Library of Congress Cataloguing in Publication data

Assessment and diagnosis of personality disorders: the International Personality Disorder
Examination (IPDE)/edited by Armand W. Loranger, Aleksandar Janca, and Norman
Sartorius.
   p.   cm.
Includes index.
ISBN 0-521-58043-9 (hardback)
1. International Personality Disorder Examination.   2. Personality disorders–Diagnosis.
I. Loranger, Armand W. (Armand Walter), 1930–   .   II. Janca, A.   III. Sartorius, N.
[DNLM: 1. Personality Disorders – diagnosis.   2. Psychiatric Status Rating Scales.
3. Personality Assessment.   WM 190 A846 1997]
RC544.A87   1997
616.85'8–dc21   96-45992 CIP
DNLM/DLC
for Library of Congress

ISBN 0 521 58043 9 hardback

TAG

Contents

Contributors

Dr Antonio Andreoli
Hopital cantonal
Unité d'urgences psychiatriques
Rue Micheli-du-crest 24
1211 Geneva 14
Switzerland
Tel: 00 41 22 372 3866; Fax: 00 41 22 372 8599

Dr Alv A. Dahl
Department of Psychiatry
University of Oslo
P.O. Box 85
Vinderen
0319 Oslo 3
Norway
Tel: 00 47 22 92 35 30; Fax: 00 47 22 49 58 61

Dr Giovanni de Girolamo
Servizio Salute Mentale
Viale Popoli 5
50123 Bologna
Italy
Tel: 00 39 51 649 1166; Fax: 00 39 51 649 2322

Dr Aleksandar Janca
Division of Mental Health and Prevention of Substance Abuse
World Health Organization
20 Avenue Appia
1211 Geneva 27
Switzerland
Tel: 00 41 22 791 3856; Fax 00 41 22 791 4160

Dr Armand W. Loranger
New York Hospital
Cornell Medical Center
Westchester Division
21 Bloomingdale Road
White Plains,
New York 10605
USA
Tel: 00 1 914 997 5922; Fax: 00 1 914 946 5859

Dr Werner Mombour
Leiter der Psychiatr. Poliklinik
Max-Planck Institut für Psychiatrie
Kraepelinstrasse 10
80804 Münich
Germany
Tel: 00 49 89 30 62 2230; Fax: 00 49 89 30 62 2200

Dr Charles Pull
Centre hospitalier de Luxembourg
Service de Neuropsychiatrie
4 rue Barblé
1210 Luxembourg
Tel: 00 352 4411 2256;4411 1706; Fax: 00 352 458 762

Dr James H. Reich
2255 North Point St.
San Francisco
CA 94123
USA
Fax: 001 415 673 2950

Dr Norman Sartorius
Department of Psychiatry
University of Geneva
1205 Geneva
Switzerland
Tel: 00 41 22 328 0078; Fax: 00 41 22 328 0079

Preface

One of the major goals of the World Health Organization's (WHO) Mental Health Programme has been the development of a common language for worldwide use by psychiatrists and other mental health professionals. The WHO/NIH Joint Project on Diagnosis and Classification of Mental Disorders, Alcohol- and Drug-related Problems is the most recent endeavour in this programme. It has developed a number of diagnostic instruments for the assessment of mental disorders in different cultures and tested them for their cross-cultural applicability, reliability and validity.[1,2]

One of these instruments, the Composite International Diagnostic Interview (CIDI),[3] is highly structured and intended for use by lay interviewers in epidemiological studies. Another, the Schedules for Clinical Assessment in Neuropsychiatry (SCAN),[4] is a semi-structured interview for use by clinicians, i.e., those capable of making independent psychiatric diagnoses. Since neither interview covers personality disorders, it was necessary to develop an instrument to assess them according to criteria in the latest classification systems.

The new instrument, the International Personality Disorder Examination (IPDE), has been developed from the Personality Disorder Examination (PDE),[5] which was modified for international use and compatibility with the International Classification of Diseases, 10th revision (ICD-10), and the American Psychiatric Association Diagnostic and Statistical Manual of Mental Disorders, fourth edition (DSM-IV). The current version of the IPDE has been produced in two modules, one for ICD-10 and one for DSM-IV criteria for personality disorders.

The IPDE was tested in a major international field trial at 14 centres in 11 countries in North America, Europe, Africa and Asia. The primary objectives were to determine its cultural acceptability, user-friendliness, interrater reliability and temporal stability. In the course of the field trial a large body of data on personality disorders in different cultures was collected. This book describes the trial, and it also addresses several related issues, including problems in the assessment of personality disorders and their rates, distribution and characteristics around the world. The book also contains the ICD-10 module of IPDE; the DSM-IV module of IPDE, without accompanying text describing its background and field trial, can be obtained from the American Psychiatric Press, Inc.

Dr Armand W. Loranger
Dr Aleksandar Janca
Dr Norman Sartorius

References

1   Sartorius, N. & Janca, A. Psychiatric assessment instruments developed by the World Health Organization. *Social Psychiatry and Psychiatric Epidemiology*, 1996; **31**: 55–69.

2   Janca, A., Ustun, T.B. & Sartorius, N. New versions of World Health Organization instruments for the assessment of mental disorders. *Acta Psychiatrica Scandinavica*, 1994; **90**: 73–83.

3   World Health Organization. *The Composite International Diagnostic Interview (CIDI)*, core version 1.1. Washington, DC: American Psychiatric Press, Inc., 1993.

4   World Health Organization. *Schedules for Clinical Assessment in Neuropsychiatry (SCAN)*, version 2.0. Washington, DC: American Psychiatric Press, Inc., 1994.

5   Loranger, A.W. *Personality Disorder Examination (PDE) Manual*. Yonkers, NY: D.V. Communications, 1988.

Acknowledgements

The IPDE was developed for the World Health Organization (WHO) by Dr. Armand W. Loranger in collaboration with the following colleagues from the international psychiatric community: Drs. Antonio Andreoli (Geneva), Peter Berger (Vienna), Peter Buchheim (Munich), S. M. Channabasavanna (Bangalore), Bina Coid (London), Alv A. Dahl (Oslo), Rene F. W. Diekstra (Leiden), Brian Ferguson (Nottingham), Lawrence B. Jacobsberg (New York), Aleksandar Janca (WHO), Werner Mombour (Munich), Yutaka Ono (Tokyo), Charles Pull (Luxembourg), Norman Sartorius (Geneva), and R. Onyango Sumba (Nairobi).

The IPDE was developed in the framework of the Joint Project on Diagnosis and Classification of Mental Disorders, Alcohol- and Drug-related Problems carried out by the WHO and US National Institutes of Health (formerly Alcohol, Drug and Mental Health Adminstration).

I   Background and Field Trial

Background

Problems in the field of personality disorders

Alv A. Dahl and Antonio Andreoli

When the World Health Organization/US Alcohol, Drug Abuse and Mental Health Administration (WHO/ADAMHA) decided to conduct the International Pilot Study of Personality Disorders (IPSPD), they entered one of the most controversial fields of mental disorders. Many psychiatrists have doubted the validity of personality disorders (PDs) and their diagnostic reliability has been found to be very low. Theories of their etiology have implicated constitution, genes, brain abnormalities, bad morals, poor environment, and disturbed psychological development. There are no generally accepted treatments for PDs, and their long-term outcome is often unknown. Since the introduction of DSM-III in 1980, however, empirical studies of PDs have flourished. The research has brought into focus many of the problems related to PDs. This chapter will describe some of them, and try to place the IPSPD and IPDE (International Personality Disorder Examination) within that context.

Basic descriptions of personality

Throughout history attempts have been made to identify the basic dimensions or categories that best define the essential similarities and differences among people. Hippocrates identified four basic temperaments based on the balance of the body fluids. The phrenologists stated that they were able to identify personality characteristics through the contour variations of the skull. Kretschmer and Sheldon described personality features based on physique, and believed that these personality types predisposed to the major mental disorders. In 1908 Heyman and Wiersma statistically analyzed the personality traits of a great number of ordinary people, and they found that personality could be described by three orthogonal factors. The study of basic personality dimensions was later promoted by Eysenck who identified three dimensions called neuroticism, extraversion, and psychoticism. Personality psychologists later expanded these to five dimensions ('the big five'), adding conscientiousness and agreeableness.[1]

Psychoanalysis introduced a general theory of personality development based on the solution of phase-specific drive conflicts during childhood. From this emerged the oral, anal, and phallic-genital personality types. As psychoanalysis progressed from a focus on drive conflicts to the study of ego functions, object relations, and self-development, a more interpersonal view was taken to describe conflicts and defects in personality functioning. For example, various interpersonal wishes and fears characterize the personality types described by Smith Benjamin.[2] Recently, a basic separation of temperament and character was proposed by Cloninger *et al.*,[3] who stated that descriptive data about individual behaviour were insufficient to permit strong preferences among alternative ways of summarizing personality traits. They proposed a general psychobiological model of personality based on three temperamental and four character dimensions.

Deviant personalities, psychopathies, and personality disorders

The problems in describing normal personality raise the fundamental question of what the difference is between normal and abnormal personality. Disorders of personality were described in the nineteenth century, along with such concepts as character, constitution, temperament, and self.[4] Pinel, in 1801, described personalities that were deviant in their emotions. Prichard, in 1835, identified patients who violated social norms as having 'moral insanity'. He raised the fundamental question, still very important in forensic psychiatry, of whether deviant personalities are mad or bad. In 1873, Koch described personality deviance in several domains as 'psychopathic inferiorities', thereby embracing the view of Morel that those with deviant personalities are inferior to normal people. The moralistic attitude towards deviant personalities was based on this assumption, and a derogatory view of patients with PD is still quite common.

From the very beginning PD was debated as a nosological entity, because of moral judgements about unacceptable personality traits, problems of their delimitation with normality, and the lack of guilt and remorse in many such patients. Because individuals with PD often did not consider themselves mentally ill, their diagnosis was less reliable than it was for many other mental disorders.

Schneider[5] proposed the view that personality traits are continuously distributed, the extreme deviations of a trait being pathological, if the individual or society suffered because of them. His 10 types of PD illustrate the fundamental arbitrariness of categorical classification of abnormal personalities. However, Schneider's classification of personality disorders influenced the International Classification of Diseases (ICD) of the WHO[6] and The Diagnostic and Statistical Manual (DSM) of the American Psychiatric Association[7] (Table 1). However, the fact that new disorders were added and deleted with each edition, confirms the validity of Lewis'[8] observation. 'It is plain that Kraepelin found the classification of PD defeating, as he frankly admits. Successive editions of his textbook show him struggling with little success, to cope with the task of shaping categories out of the rich variety of human character and conduct. His efforts and his failure are characteristic examples of the frustration which besets students of personality when they aim at precision.'

Table 1. *Classification of personality disorders*

Schneider (1923)	ICD-10 (1993)	DSM-III-R (1987)
Depressive	–	–
Hyperthymic	–	Cyclothymia*
Fanatical	Paranoid	Paranoid
	Emotionally unstable:	
Explosive	Impulsive type	Explosive*
Labile	Borderline type	Borderline
Affectionless	Dissocial	Antisocial
Insecure:		
sensitive	Anxious (avoidant)	Avoidant
anancastic	Anankastic	Obsessive-compulsive
Asthenic	Hypochondriasis*	Hypochondriasis*
Attention-seeking	Histrionic	Histrionic
–	Schizoid	Schizoid
–	Dependent	Dependent
–	–	Schizotypal
–	–	Narcissistic
–	–	Passive aggressive

*Located elsewhere in the classification

The relation to normal personality

Abnormal personality traits exist in milder forms in normal individuals. If the traits manifest themselves as inflexible responses to a broad range of personal and social situations and result in considerable personal distress or social disruption, they are called PD. They represent extreme or significant deviations from the way in which the average individual in a given culture perceives, thinks, feels, and relates to others. They are thus only quantitatively and not qualitatively different from normal personality. However, the border between normal and abnormal personalities is difficult to draw.

The relation to culture and sex

Cultural diversity is a characteristic of human nature. Behavioural patterns considered normal in one culture are seen as deviant in another. To identify behavioural patterns that are deviant in all cultures is very difficult. The PDs primarily reflect the views of Western European and North American psychiatry and they may not be equally applicable in other cultures. Role expectations and behaviour, also differ considerably between the sexes. Problems may arise if psychiatry defines personality deviance without considering social role expectations.

Unknown personality traits and the use of informants

Many individuals may be unaware of some of their personality traits and behavioural patterns. Therefore, an individual often can only provide limited information about him or herself. He/she may also consciously try to deny certain socially undesirable personality traits. These problems can partially be solved by interviewing an informant who knows the individual well, but this is still not a standard procedure in the evaluation of PD. Sometimes informants describe PD-pathology that patients deny.[9] When the accounts of the subject and the informant deviate, which source of information is more valid? A method of integrating information from such discrepant reports is needed.

Separate axis and diagnostic criteria

The DSM of Mental Disorders, Third Edition (DSM-III)[7] published by the American Psychiatric Association in 1980 made two innovations of major importance for the study of PDs. They were placed on a separate axis (Axis II), and explicit criteria provided guidelines for the diagnosis of each of the 11 PDs. The introduction of diagnostic criteria stimulated empirical research on the reliability of PDs and the optimal diagnostic criteria.

In DSM-III, PDs were defined by both monothetic and polythetic sets of criteria. Monothetic requires that all criteria be fulfilled, while polythetic requires patients to meet a certain number of the total criteria set, thus allowing some variation in the symptoms of patients with the same disorder. In DSM-III-R[7] all PDs were defined by sets of polythetic criteria. The number of criteria found in a patient can also be used as a dimensional rating of that PD. For each disorder a cut-off level for a positive diagnosis has been arbitrarily set. It has been shown[9] that the interrater reliability of PD diagnoses is higher in samples of patients with more prototypical forms of a disorder. Following the publication of DSM-III there was considerable debate about the reliability and validity of certain criteria,[10] and revisions were made in DSM-III-R and DSM-IV.

'State–Trait' problems

When DSM-III separated the mental disorders into two axes, Axis II was reserved for disorders that, 'all share the features of generally having an onset in childhood or adolescence and usually persisting in a stable form (without periods of remission or exacerbation) into adult life. With only a few exceptions, these features are not present for Axis I disorders'.[7] However, sometimes certain Axis I disorders may begin early in life and produce changes in personality. Some PDs may also predispose to Axis I disorders. Some Axis I disorders change behaviour temporarily, and in a cross-sectional evaluation it is often difficult to determine if the patient's behaviour represents longstanding personality traits or symptoms of a current Axis I disorder, that will disappear with improvement in the disorder (state). Confounding trait and state seems to be one of the main reasons clinicians sometimes over-diagnose PDs. They often do not adequately explore the duration of a behavioural pattern. Self-report instruments for diagnosing PDs are especially sensitive to this artifact, which may explain the high proportion of false positive PD diagnoses with such instruments.

The IPDE requires a duration of at least five years, and onset before the age of 25 for abnormal personality traits. Loranger et al.[11] demonstrated that the state–trait problem was negligible when the Personality Disorder Examination (PDE) was used by experienced clinicians. But Zimmerman, in his review of PD studies[9] found that PD examinations during acute psychiatric states gave higher rates than after normalization of the Axis I disorder. If possible, a diagnosis of PD should be postponed if the patient is psychotic or severely depressed or anxious. Since PDs concern a patient's long-term functioning, the PD diagnosis should be stable over time. Test–retest reliability studies of PDs show a falloff in reliability from initial to short-term and long-term examination.[9]

Categories and dimensions

In practice many patients receive a diagnosis of several PDs at the same examination. This diagnostic overlap creates problems in defining homogeneous groups in psychiatric research. Although DSM-III-R outlined three clusters of PDs, the eccentric, dramatic, and anxious, diagnostic overlap is often found both within and across these clusters. One cause of diagnostic overlap is that similar diagnostic criteria are used to define several PDs. Multiple PD diagnoses are also caused by the use of arbitrary categories, which may not correspond to latent constructs or personality dimensions. In DSM-IV[12] the overlap in criteria has been reduced to some extent.

DSM and ICD have adopted a categorical classification system. They provide simplified abstractions which are easy to communicate, but important information about the patient is subsequently lost. A dimensional approach to PD classification, which locates patients along a set of dimensions, has obvious advantages, but none have been used yet in any nosology. Although a dimensional approach provides more information, it is more difficult to communicate. There also seems to be a lack of agreement regarding which dimensions to include, but this problem now seems closer to a solution.[13]

Progress in the field of psychiatric diagnoses

Although validation of psychiatric diagnoses is generally lacking, considerable progress has been made since the late 1980s.[14] Diagnostic criteria for mental disorders have made diagnoses more reliable. This is particularly so, when used in combination with structured psychiatric interviews. Although several PD instruments have been developed recently, their transcultural validity is virtually unknown.[15] Statistics have been developed which give a meaningful description of interrater reliability,[16] and with the use of videotaped interviews patients can be diagnosed by trained clinicians all around the world. Because of this methodological progress, a study such as the ISPSD was indicated. Its objectives were to: determine the feasibilty of using a standardized semi-structured interview (IPDE) to identify and diagnose PDs in different cultures; determine the interrater reliability of the IPDE in its various language versions; and investigate selected aspects of assessment, such as temporal stability. All of these objectives are essential to progress in the field of PD.

References

1   McCrae, R.R. & Costa, Jr., P.T. *Personality in Adulthood.* New York: Guilford, 1990.
2   Smith Benjamin, L. *Interpersonal Diagnosis and Treatment of Personality Disorders.* New York: Guilford, 1993.
3   Cloninger, C.R., Svrakic, D.M. & Przybeck, T.R. A psychobiological model of temperament and character. *Archives of General Psychiatry*, 1993; **50**: 975–90.
4   Berrios, G.E. European views on personality disorders: a conceptual history. *Comprehensive Psychiatry*, 1993; **34**: 14–30.
5   Schneider, K. *Psychopathic Personalities.* London: Cassell, 1950.
6   World Health Organization. *International Statistical Classification of Diseases and Related Health Problems*, 10th revision. Geneva: World Health Organisation, 1992.
7   American Psychiatric Association. *Diagnostic and Statistical Manual of Mental Disorders*, 3rd revised edn. Washington, DC, American Psychiatric Press 1987.
8   Lewis, A. Psychopathic personality: a most elusive category. *Psychological Medicine*, 1974; **4**: 133–40.
9   Zimmerman, M. Diagnosing personality disorders. A review of issues and research methods. *Archives of General Psychiatry*, 1994; **51**: 225–45.
10 Livesley, W.J. & Jackson, D.N. Guidelines for developing, evaluating, and revising the classification of personality disorders. *Journal of Nervous and Mental Disease*, 1992; **180**: 609–18.
11 Loranger, A.W., Lenzenweger, M.F., Gartner, A.F., Susman, V.L. *et al.* Trait-state artifacts and the diagnosis of personality disorders. *Archives of General Psychiatry*, 1991; **48**: 720–8.
12 American Psychiatric Association. *Diagnostic and Statistical Manual of Mental Disorders*, revised 4th edn. Washington, DC, American Psychiatric Press 1994.
13 Widiger, T.A. Personality disorder dimensional models proposed for DSM-IV. *Journal of Personality Disorders*,1991; **5**: 386–98.
14 Kendell, R.E. Clinical validity. *Psychological Medicine*, 1989; **19**: 45–55.
15 Reich, J.H. Instruments measuring DSM-III and DSM-III-R personality disorders. *Journal Personality Disorders*, 1987; **1**: 220–40.
16 Bartko, J.J. & Carpenter, W. On the methods and theory of reliability. *Journal Nervous and Mental Diseases*, 1976; **163**: 307–17.

Review of diagnostic instruments for the assessment of personality disorders

Armand W. Loranger

This chapter is intended to acquaint the reader with most of the instruments specifically designed to diagnose the personality disorders (PDs). The review makes no pretense at completeness. Preference is given to interviews and inventories that have also been used by investigators other than the developers themselves. The International Personality Disorder Examination (IPDE) is not included, since most of this volume (see Part II) is devoted to it. The account is mainly descriptive rather than analytical. For more of the latter, the interested reader will find Zimmerman's recent review especially informative.[1]

There is an axiom in psychometrics that the more closely a test samples the criterion it attempts to predict, the more valid it is likely to be. Historically, the identification and delineation of PDs has emerged primarily from clinical observation. Therefore, it should not be surprising if diagnoses based on semistructured clinical interviews approximate clinical diagnoses more than those based on self-administered inventories. The obvious limitation of the latter is their inability to provide the observations, cross-examination, and judgement of the experienced clinician. Except for the dementias and mental retardation, there is nothing in the history of clinical psychological tests to warrant their being viewed as a close approximation to a psychiatric diagnosis.

Self-administered tests, however, may be valuable as economical screening devices. The literature suggests that personality disorder inventories are especially prone to false-positive diagnoses.[2] Of course this is precisely what one expects from a screening instrument, where the main concern is to guard against an intolerable number of false-negatives. Because dimensional information is often used to supplement categorical PD diagnoses, inventories may also prove useful in estimating the extent to which an individual shares certain maladaptive traits with those who fulfill the categorical requirements for a particular type of PD. The estimates, however, are likely to be no more than moderately correlated with dimensional assessments based on semistructured clinical interviews.

Personality Disorder Interviews

Diagnostic Interview for Borderlines (DIB)

In the years immediately preceding the appearance of DSM-III, Gunderson and his colleagues developed an interview for the diagnosis of borderline personality disorder.[3] The DIB was based on criteria quite similar to those ultimately adopted by the DSM-III. In its revised form (DIB-R)[4] it consists of 186 questions divided into four sections: affect, cognition, impulse action patterns, and interpersonal relationships. The information obtained from the questions is used to rate 22 statements that describe important features of borderline personality disorder. The scores are then algorithmically scaled to yield a total score of 0 to 10, with a recommended cutoff score of 8 required for the diagnosis. Typically, the interview takes between 45 minutes and 1 hour to complete. In the 1980s the original DIB was used in a large number of research investigations of borderline disorder. There is now a considerable literature and, not surprisingly, it shows varying agreement with clinical and other methods of diagnosing borderline disorder.

Structured Interview for DSM-III-R Personality Disorders (SIDP-R)

The revised form of the SIDP-R, developed by Pfohl and colleagues at the University of Iowa, is organized into 17 topically oriented sections, each containing about 10 questions.[5] At the end of every section there is a list of those DSM-III-R criteria that are to be rated as: not present (0), moderately present (1), or severely present (2), on the basis of the subject's responses to the questions in the section. Brief descriptors serve as anchors in rating, and a score of either 1 or 2 is considered evidence that the criterion has been met. At the end of the interview there is a summary rating form with the criteria listed by PD. The interview usually takes between one and a half and two hours.

When feasible the interviewer is expected to use information from other sources, including an informant interview based on some of the same questions. The authors have reported poor agreement between patient and informant regarding whether or not a PD is present (kappa=.13).[6] Other than the judgement of the interviewer, there are no specific guidelines for dealing with such conflicting information. Published data on interrater agreement in scoring the original version of the SIDP indicate that, in general, the reliability is quite satisfactory and comparable to that obtained with similar interviews.[7]

Structured Clinical Interview for DSM-III-R (SCID-II)

The SCID-II is a personality disorder module of the popular SCID,[8] a diagnostic interview developed by Spitzer and colleagues that is intended to help the clinician make most DSM-III-R diagnoses. It differs from the main Axis I SCID interview, as well as from other PD interviews, in that it is preceded by a 113-item personality questionnaire concerning the Axis II criteria. The purpose of this is to save interview time. Ordinarily the patient is interviewed only about those criteria that are acknowledged on the questionnaire. The interview itself is organized on a disorder by disorder basis, rather than around certain topics or domains of behaviour. The examiner is expected to use follow-up questions as needed and is encouraged to use other sources of information as well. As one proceeds through the interview, the individual criteria are scored as: absent (1), subthreshold (2), or threshold (3). The SCID-II, along with the parent SCID, has been the subject of a multicentre study of interrater reliability. Detailed results have yet to be published, but they are reported to be similar to those with the SIDP and the IPDE.[1] It will be particularly important to determine the extent to which false-negative diagnoses may be expected as a consequence of the questionnaire-interview format that is unique to the SCID-II.

Personality Assessment Schedule (PAS)

The PAS which is in its fifth revision, was developed in England by Tyrer and his colleagues[9-11] and has received limited use elsewhere. The interview inquires about 24 personality characteristics that are rated on a 9-point scale at the conclusion. Preference is given to interviewing informants rather than patients because they are thought to be in a better position to assess the social disruption caused by abnormal traits and to be free of the distortion produced by the current mental state. The interview is said to take about one hour to complete if both patient and informant are interviewed.

The 24 personality attributes assessed by the schedule are pessimism, worthlessness, optimism, lability, anxiousness, suspiciousness, introspection, shyness, aloofness, sensitivity, vulnerability, irritability, impulsiveness, aggression, callousness, irresponsibility, childishness, resourcelessness, dependence, submissiveness, conscientiousness, rigidity, eccentricity, and hypochondriasis. The authors used a cluster analysis of their data to identify four major types of abnormal personality: sociopathic, passive-dependent, anankastic, and schizoid. Nine subsidiary categories also emerged: explosive (impulsive), sensitive aggressive, histrionic, asthenic, anxious, paranoid, hypochondriacal, dysthymic, and avoidant.

Interrater agreement in rating the 24 attributes on a dimensional scale is reported to be generally good, as has that for the diagnosis of a PD *per se*. Poor agreement, however, has been found between patients and informants, and some studies have used an arbitrary and complicated set of guidelines to determine which information to use.

The 24 personality dimensions on the PAS are neither described in detail nor defined by specific criteria. They are rated according to the degree of social impairment they produce. This is a departure from DSM-III-R and ICD-10, which include subjective distress as well as social impairment in the definition of a personality disorder, although both are not required for a diagnosis. The PAS mandates social impairment and is not directly concerned with subjective distress. The assumption is that if subjective distress is high enough to be indicative of a personality disorder, then marked social impairment will be present. The PAS also follows a hierarchical system of diagnosis that identifies the disorder with the greatest social impairment as the primary one. Although the PAS was not developed to assess the PDs in DSM-III-R or ICD-10, it does provide algorithms for making diagnoses in those systems. It is not known, however, whether the algorithms will identify the same cases as those interviews based on the criteria themselves.

Standardized Assessment of Personality (SAP)

The SAP[12] is a short semistructured interview developed by Pilgrim and Mann, and designed for use with a relative or close friend of a patient. It takes 10–15 minutes to administer. The informant is asked to describe the patient's personality prior to illness, and a series of probes explores specific areas of personality. Although it claims to assess PDs in the ICD-10 and DSM-III-R classification systems, it does not systematically survey the more than 100 criteria on which those two systems are based. It has had limited use so far, other than by its developers.

Personality Disorder Inventories

Millon Clinical Multiaxial Inventory (MCMI)

The MCMI is unique in that it is based on the author's own theory of personality and psychopathology and also claims to be congruent with the

DSM-III-R nosology. It is not considered suitable for use with normals. The latest version (MCMI-II)[13] consists of 175 true–false items aggregated in 20 clinical scales. These in turn are organized into three broad categories: persistent personality features, current symptom states, and levels of pathology. Norms for the test are based on several groups of normal subjects and numerous clinical samples. They include base rate scores calculated from prevalence data. The claim that it maps the domain of DSM-III Axis II has been challenged and remains to be demonstrated.[14-18] Although more research on this subject needs to be done, efforts so far to establish a correspondence between the MCMI and the clinical diagnosis of PDs have been disappointing.[19-22]

Personality Diagnostic Questionnaire (PDQ-R)

In its revised form the PDQ-R is a 189-item true–false questionnaire developed by Hyler and associates.[23] The content is keyed to the DSM-III-R personality disorders. One or more items are devoted to each Axis II criterion, and the wording is close to the criteria. For example, the borderline criterion, 'Inappropriate, intense anger or lack of control of anger,' is assessed by these two statements: 'I rarely get so angry that I lose control' (false) and 'I've often gotten into more real physical fights than most people' (true). A borderline diagnosis is given when the respondent answers at least one of the items that sample each of the five or more criteria required for the diagnosis in the DSM-III-R.

As with the MCMI, studies have generally found a poor correspondence between the PDQ and personality diagnoses made by clinicians with and without semistructured interviews.[24-27]

Tridimensional Personality Questionnaire (TPQ)

The TPQ,[28] developed by Cloninger is a 100-item self-report inventory that measures three major personality dimensions: novelty seeking, harm avoidance, and reward dependence. The inventory is based on a theoretical biosocial model that integrates neuroanatomical and neurophysiological constructs with learning styles and three personality dimensions. Normative data are based on a US sample of 1019 adults. The TPQ is available in a number of languages.

Novelty seeking has four subscales: exploratory excitability vs stoic rigidity (9 items), impulsiveness vs reflection (8 items), extravagance vs reserve (7 items), and disorderliness vs regimentation (10 items). Harm avoidance has four subscales: anticipatory worry vs uninhibited optimism (10 items), fear of uncertainty vs confidence (7 items), shyness with strangers vs gregariousness (7 items), and fatigability and asthenia vs vigor (10 items). Reward dependence has four subscales: sentimentality vs insensitiveness (5 items), persistence vs irresoluteness (9 items), attachment vs detachment (11 items) and dependence vs independence (5 items).

Temperament and Character Inventory (TCI)

As might have been anticipated, Cloninger discovered that certain temperament types occurred more frequently with some PDs. However, contrary to his original expectation, individuals with extreme temperament profiles on the TPQ did not necessarily have PDs; indeed some were well adapted normals. Consequently, Cloninger subsequently invoked the additional role of 'character' traits. According to his revised theory[29] temperament, which now includes a fourth dimension, persistence, determines the type of PD, but character determines whether there will be a PD. The 226-item true–false TCI, enlarges the scope of the TPQ to measure the acquired self-concept character traits of self-directedness, cooperatives, and self-transcendence. Preliminary data[30] suggest that each type of PD in DSM-III-R is associated with a unique profile of scores on the TCI. Although the test has been promoted as an efficient guide to diagnosis and treatment, information is not yet available regarding the sensitivity and specificity of the TCI in identifying the individual DSM-III-R personality disorders, when they are diagnosed by clinicians using semistuctured interviews.

References

1 Zimmerman, M. Diagnosing personality disorders: a review of issues and methods. *Archives of General Psychiatry*, 1994; **51**: 225–45.

2 Loranger, A.W. Are current self-report and interview measures adequate for epidemiological studies of personality disorders? *Journal of Personality Disorders*, 1992; **6**: 313–25.

3 Gunderson, J.G. & Kolb, J.E. The Diagnostic Interview for Borderlines. *American Journal of Psychiatry*, 1981; **138**: 896.

4 Zanarini, M.C., Gunderson, J.G., Frankenburg, F.R. & Chauncey, D.L. The revised Diagnostic Interview for Borderlines: Discriminating BPD from other Axis II disorders. *Journal of Personality Disorders*, 1989; **3**: 10.

5 Pfohl, B., Blum, N., Zimmerman, M. & Stangl, D. Structured Interview for

DSM-III-R Personality SIDP-R, draft edition. Iowa City, Department of Psychiatry, University of Iowa, April 27, 1989.

6 Zimmerman, M., Pfohl, B., Coryell, W. *et al.* Diagnosing personality disorder in depressed patients. A comparison of patient and informant interviews. *Archives of General Psychiatry,* 1988; **45**: 733.

7 Stangl, D., Pfohl, B., Zimmerman, M. *et al.* A structured interview for the DSM-III personality disorders: A preliminary report. *Archives of General Psychiatry,* 1985; **42**: 591.

8 Spitzer, R.L., Williams, J.B.W., Gibbon, M. & First, M. *User's Guide for the Structured Clinical Interview for DSM-III-R.* Washington, DC: American Psychiatric Association Press, 1990.

9 Tyrer, P. *Personality Disorders: Diagnosis, Management and Course.* Boston: Wright, 1988.

10 Tyrer, P., Strauss, J. & Cicchetti, D. Temporal reliability of personality in psychiatric patients. *Psychological Medicine,* 1983; **13**: 393.

11 Tyrer, P., Cicchetti, D.V., Casey, P.R. *et al.* Cross-national reliability study of a schedule for assessing personality disorders. *Journal of Nervous and Mental Disease,* 1984; **172**: 718.

12 Pilgrim, J. & Mann, A. Use of the ICD-10 version of the Standardized Assessment of Personality to determine the prevalence of personality disorder in psychiatric patients. *Psychological Medicine,* 1990; **20**: 985–91.

13 Millon T. *Manual for the MCMI-II,* 2nd edn. Minneapolis: National Computer Systems, 1987.

14 Widiger, T.A., Williams, J.B.W., Spitzer, R.L. & Frances, A. The MCMI as a measure of DSM-III. *Journal of Personality Assessment,* 1985; **49**: 366.

15 Widiger, T.A., Williams, J.B.W., Spitzer, R.L. & Frances, A. The MCMI and DSM-III: A brief rejoinder to Millon. *Journal of Personality Assessment,* 1986; **50**: 198.

16 Widiger, T.A. & Sanderson, C. The convergent and discriminant validity of the MCMI as a measure of the DSM-III personality disorders. *Journal of Personality Assessment,* 1987; **51**: 228.

17 Millon, T. The MCMI provides a good assessment of DSM-III disorders: The MCMI-II will prove even better. *Journal of Personality Assessment,* 1985; **49**: 379.

18 Millon, T. The MCMI and DSM-III: Further commentaries. *Journal of Personality Assessment,* 1986; **50**: 205.

19 Reich, J.H., Noyes, R. & Troughton, E. Comparison of three DSM-III personality disorder instruments. In *Conference on the Millon Clinical Inventories (MCMI, MBHI, MAPI).* Minneapolis: National Computer Systems, 1987.

20 Wetzler, S. & Dubro, A. Diagnosis of personality disorders by the Millon Clinical Multiaxial Inventory. *Journal of Nervous and Mental Disease,* 1990; **178**: 261.

21 Piersma, H.L. The MCMI as a measure of DSM-III Axis II diagnoses: An empirical comparison. *Journal of Clinical Psychology,* 1987; **43**: 479.

22   Repko, G.R. & Cooper, R. The diagnosis of personality disorder: A comparison of MMPI profile, Millon Inventory, and clinical judgment. *Journal of Clinical Psychology,* 1985; **41**: 867.

23   Hyler, S.E. & Rieder, R.O. *PDQ-R Personality Questionnaire.* New York: New York State Psychiatric Institute, July 15, 1986.

24   Hurt. S.W., Hyler, S.E., Frances, A. *et al.* Assessing borderline personality disorder with self-report, clinical interview or semistructured interview. *American Journal of Psychiatry,* 1984; **141**: 1228.

25   Hyler, S.E., Rieder, R.O., Williams, J.B.W. *et al.* A comparison of clinical and self-report diagnoses of DSM-III personality disorders in 552 patients. *Comprehensive Psychiatry,* 1989; **30**: 170.

26   Pfohl, B., Barrash, J., True, B. & Alexander, B. Failure of two Axis I measures to predict medication noncompliance among hypertensive patients. *Journal of Personality Disorders,* 1989; **3**: 45.

27   Dubro, A., Wetzler, S. & Kahn, M.W. A comparison of three self-report questionnaires for the diagnosis of DSM-III personality disorders. *Journal of Personality Disorders,* 1988; **2**: 256.

28   Cloninger, C.R. A systematic method for clinical description and classification of personality variants. *Archives of General Psychiatry,* 1987; **44**: 573–88.

29   Cloninger, C.R., Svrakic, D.M. & Przybeck, T.R. A psychobiological model of temperament and character. *Archives of General Psychiatry,* 1993; **50**: 975–90.

30   Svrakic, D.M., Whitehead, C., Przybeck, T.R. & Cloninger, C.R. Differential diagnosis of personality disorders by the seven-factor model of temperament and character. *Archives of General Psychiatry,* 1993; **50**: 991–99.

Epidemiology of DSM-III personality disorders in the community and in clinical populations

James H. Reich and Giovanni de Girolamo

Although the early Greek philosophers wondered about the influence of personality on health, it is only recently that the epidemiology of personality disorders (PDs) has begun to be scientifically investigated. This is because we have now developed a number of standardized instruments to assess personality and PD in an empirical fashion. The first comprehensive epidemiologic reviews in the English language have only been published since the mid-1980s.[1-4] The need for the epidemiological investigation of PD seems justified for several reasons: firstly, as seen in the most recent epidemiological surveys, PDs are frequent and have been found in different countries and sociocultural settings; secondly, PDs can seriously impair the life of the affected individual and can be highly disruptive to societies, communities, and families; thirdly, personality status is often a major predictive variable in determining the outcome of psychiatric disorders and the response to treatment.[5,6]

In this chapter we review the main epidemiological literature on PDs up to the end of 1993, focusing mainly on studies employing DSM-III or DSM-III-related measures of personality. Firstly community prevalence studies of PD will be reviewed. We then look at the prevalence of individual PDs in the community. Finally, we consider PDs in psychiatric populations. Many of the DSM-III categories of PD have counterparts in the ICD-10 classification; however, when this chapter was being written, there were no studies yet which directly employed ICD-10 criteria. For those interested in the literature prior to DSM-III and ICD-10, Neugebauer et al.[7] reviewed 20 epidemiological psychiatric studies carried out in Europe and North America since 1950. They found an average prevalence rate for PD of 7%. However, their estimate included alcoholism and drug abuse among the PDs. A few years later Perry and Vaillant[8] suggested that between 5 and 15% of the adult population can be expected to manifest PDs.

Four recently published studies ascertained the prevalence rate of PD in community samples, and used assessment instruments specific for PD.[9–12] They will be briefly reviewed separately.

In a random sample of 200 people selected from urban and rural communities and assessed with the Personality Assessment Schedule (PAS), a PD was found in 26 subjects (13%).[9] Explosive PD was the most common type. There were no differences between urban and rural samples, or between men and women among the 16 (8%) identified as psychiatric cases on the Present State Examination (PSE), more than half of whom also had a PD. Social functioning was worse in those with PD than in those with a normal personality, with no significant differences among the different categories of PD.

Maier et al.[10] surveyed an unscreened sample of 109 families for lifetime diagnoses of both Axis I disorders and PD. Among 447 subjects who were personally interviewed with the Schedule for Affective Disorders and Schizophrenia-Lifetime Version (SADS-L) and the Structured Clinical Interview for DSM-III-R (SCID-II), they found rates of PD comparable to the other studies. The rate among males was 9.9% and among females 10.5%, and it was higher in younger than in older subjects. Significant associations between current Axis I disorders and PD were observed, in particular anxiety disorders with avoidant PD, and affective disorders with borderline PD.

In a community sample of 235 adults surveyed with a self-administered instrument, the Personality Diagnostic Questionnaire (PDQ), 26 were diagnosed as having a PD, yielding an age-adjusted prevalence of 11.1%.[11] A history of alcohol abuse, poor employment, and marital problems was more common in the group with PDs. The age and sex distribution of the DSM-III personality cluster traits was also assessed.[13] Traits in the schizoid cluster were not associated with age, while those in the dramatic and the anxious clusters were. Women aged 31 to 40 and men aged 18 to 30 had the highest rate of PDs. Women aged 31 to 40 had a higher mean number of traits than their male counterparts, and also a corresponding increase in impairment.

In a study by Zimmerman and Coryell, 697 relatives of psychiatric patients and healthy controls who were interviewed with the Structured Interview for Personality Disorders (SIPD) also took the PDQ.[12] More had a PD according to the interview than the questionnaire (13.5% vs 10.33%). Schizotypal, histrionic, antisocial and passive-aggressive were the most frequent diagnoses from the SIDP, while dependent PD and multiple diagnoses were more frequent using the PDQ. One conclusion from this study that is especially relevant to the present review, is that questionnaire and interview assessments of PD generally show a poor concordance. Therefore, the type of assessment can strongly affect the rate of a disorder.

To summarize, although different investigators have used different instruments and populations, the prevalence of PD ranged from 10.3% to 13.5%, a highly consistent prevalence rate of PD in the community. The rate seems to vary with age, with a slight decrease in older age-groups. Urban populations and lower socioeconomic groups showed higher rates. Although the sex ratio is different for specific types of PD, the overall rates of PD are about equal for the two sexes.

Community epidemiological studies of specified personality disorders

Table 1 lists the prevalence rates for specific PDs. The majority of the estimates come from three studies.[10,12,13] In addition, data on the prevalence of some specified PDs have been reported by Baron et al.,[14] who assessed 750 first-degree relatives of chronic schizophrenics (n = 376) and normal control probands (n = 374). They administered the subjects the SADS, the Schedule for Interviewing Borderlines (SIB) and additional items to diagnose other specific PDs, for which the two interview schedules did not provide adequate coverage.

Paranoid

Reich et al.[15] and Zimmerman and Coryell[12] have found comparable rates, ranging from 0.4% to 0.8%, while Maier et al.[10] found slightly higher rates, 1.8%. Baron et al.[14] found a significantly higher rate of paranoid PD among relatives of schizophrenic probands (7.3%) than among relatives of control probands (2.7%). This disorder seems to be more frequent among the members of the lower social classes.

Schizoid

Maier et al.,[10] Reich et al.,[15] and Zimmerman and Coryell[12] reported rates ranging from 0.4% to 0.9%. Baron et al.[14] reported a rate of 1.6% among relatives of schizophrenic probands and to no cases among relatives of control probands.

Schizotypal

Reich et al.[15] and Zimmerman and Coryell[12] reported rates of 3.0% and 5.6% respectively, while Maier et al.[10] found a substantially lower rate

Table 1. *Prevalence rates of specified personality disorders (PDs) in epidemiologic surveys or in relatives*

Type of PD	Author and year of publication (Ref. no.)	Country	Sample size	Assessment method	PD prevalence rate (%)
Paranoid	Baron et al., 1985 (14)	USA	376* 374**	SIB, SADS	7.3* 2.7**
	Maier et al., 1992 (10)	Germany	447	SCID	1.8
	Reich et al., 1989b (15)	USA	235	PDQ	0.8
	Zimmerman & Coryell, 1990 (12)	USA	697	PDQ SIPD	0.4 0.4
Schizoid	Baron et al., 1985 (14)	USA	376* 374**	SIB, SADS	1.6* 0**
	Maier et al., 1992 (10)	Germany	447	SCID	0.4
	Reich et al., 1989b (15)	USA	235	PDQ	0.8
	Zimmerman & Coryell, 1990 (12)	USA	697	PDQ SIPD	0.9 0.7
Schizotypal	Baron et al., 1985 (14)	USA	376* 374**	SIB, SADS	14.6* 2.1**
	Maier et al., 1992 (10)	Germany	447	SCID	0.6
	Reich et al., 1989b (15)	USA	235	PDQ	5.1
	Zimmerman & Coryell, 1990 (12)	USA	697	PDQ SIPD3	5.6 3.0
Histrionic	Maier et al., 1992 (10)	Germany	447	SCID	1.3
	Nestadt et al., 1990 (16)	USA	810	SPE	2.1
	Reich et al., 1989b (15)	USA	235	PDQ	2.1

Table 1. (*contd.*)

Type of PD	Author and year of publication (Ref. no.)	Country	Sample size	Assessment method	PD prevalence rate (%)
	Zimmerman & Coryell, 1990 (12)	USA	697	PDQ	2.7
				SIPD	3.0
Narcissistic	Maier *et al.*, 1992 (10)	Germany	447	SCID	0
	Reich *et al.*, 1989b (15)	USA	235	PDQ	0.4
	Zimmerman & Coryell, 1990 (12)	USA	697	PDQ	0.4
				SIPD	0
Borderline	Baron *et al.*, 1985 (14)	USA	376*	SIB, SADS	1.9*
			374**		1.6**
	Maier *et al.*, 1992 (10)	Germany	447	SCID	1.1
	Reich *et al.*, 1989b (15)	USA	235	PDQ	1.3
	Swartz *et al.*, 1990 (18)	USA	1,541	DIB/DIS	1.8
	Zimmerman & Coryell, 1990 (12)	USA	697	PDQ	4.6
				SIPD	1.7
	Weissman & Myers, 1980 (17)	USA	511	SADS-L	0.2
Avoidant	Baron *et al.*, 1985 (14)	USA	376*	SIB, SADS	1.6*
			374**	0**	
	Maier *et al.*, 1992 (10)	Germany	447	SCID	1.1
	Reich *et al.*, 1989b (15)	USA	235	PDQ	0
	Zimmerman & Coryell, 1990 (12)	USA	697	PDQ	0.4
				SIPD	1.3

	Study	Country	N	Instrument	%
Dependent	Baron et al., 1985 (14)	USA	376* / 374**	SIB, SADS	0.3* / 0**
	Maier et al., 1992 (10)	Germany	447	SCID	1.6
	Reich et al., 1989b (15)	USA	235	PDQ	5.1
	Zimmerman & Coryell, 1990 (12)	USA	697	PDQ	6.7
				SIPD	1.7
Compulsive	Maier et al., 1992 (10)	Germany	447	SCID	2.2
	Nestadt et al., 1991 (16)	USA	759	SPE	1.7
	Reich et al., 1989b (15)	USA	235	PDQ	6.4
	Zimmerman & Coryell, 1990 (12)	USA	697	PDQ	4.0
				SIPD	1.7
Passive-Aggressive	Maier et al., 1992 (10)	Germany	447	SCID	1.8
	Reich et al., 1989b (15)	USA	235	PDQ	0
	Zimmerman & Coryell, 1990 (12)	USA	697	PDQ	0.4
				SIPD	3.0

Adapted in part from Weissman, 1991

* First-degree relatives of chronic schizophrenics. ** Normal control probands. Abbreviations: SIB, Schedule for Interviewing Borderlines; SADS, Schedule for Affective Disorders and Schizophrenia; SCID, Structured Clinical Interview for DSM-III-R; PDQ, Personality Diagnostic Questionnaire; SIPD, Structured Interview for Personality Disorders; SPE, Standardized Psychiatric Examination; SADS-L, Schedule for Affective Disorders and Schizophrenia – Lifetime Version; DIB, Diagnostic Interview for Borderlines; DIS, Diagnostic Interview Schedule.

(0.6%). The rates obtained with similar instruments such as the PDQ are strikingly similar despite differences in sample size, characteristics, and response rates. In the study by Baron et al.,[14] schizotypal PD was remarkably more common among relatives of schizophrenic probands (14.6%) than among relatives of control probands (2.1%). This result provides additional support for the specific relationship between schizophrenia and schizotypal PD.

Histrionic

A study by Nestadt et al.,[16] carried out at the Baltimore (USA) site of the Epidemiological Catchment Area Program (ECA), ascertained the prevalence of histrionic PD in the community. The authors found a prevalence of 2.1% in the general population, with virtually identical rates in men and women. No significant differences were found in terms of race and education, but the prevalence was significantly higher among separated and divorced persons. Moreover, 17% of the women with histrionic PD also had a depressive disorder, an increased rate of suicide attempts, and a fourfold increase in utilization of medical services. It should be noted that the study derived the diagnosis from instruments not originally intended to diagnose personality disorders.

Narcissistic

Reich et al.[15] and Zimmerman and Coryell,[12] using the PDQ, found identical rates (0.4%) of narcissistic disorder. No cases were found by Maier et al.[10] with the SCID, or Zimmerman and Coryell[12] with the SIPD.

Borderline

Borderline and antisocial, have been the most studied PDs. In 1975 Weissman and Myers,[17] in a survey carried out in New Haven (USA) among a sample of 511 subjects using the SADS-L and RDC, reported a rate of only 0.2%. However, this rate was derived from an instrument not designed to measure DSM-III borderline PD.

Reich et al.[15] reported a rate of 1.3% of borderline PD with the PDQ. Zimmerman and Coryell[12] obtained rates of 1.7% with the SIPD and 4.6% with the PDQ. The rate of 1.7% was similar to that (1.1%) reported by Maier et al.[10] Borderlines, compared to those with other PDs, exhibited higher rates of alcohol, tobacco use, phobic disorders, suicide attempts, and schizophrenia. The borderlines were also younger and less likely to be married. Those who did marry were likely to be divorced or separated.

Swartz et al.[18] carried out a study among 1541 community subjects (19–55 years of age) at the North Carolina site of the ECA, using a diagnostic algorithm derived from the Diagnostic Interview Schedule (DIS). They found a rate of 1.8%, and the disorder was significantly more common among females, the widowed, and the unmarried. There was a trend towards an increase in the diagnosis in younger, non-white, urban, and poorer respondents. The highest rates were found in the 19 to 34 age range, with the rates declining with age. All border-line respondents had also a DIS DSM-III, Axis I lifetime diagnosis. The borderline group included high users of such services, with 50% having had contact with out-patient mental health services in the previous six months. However, the borderlines did not use general medical services more than the total population, and they had similar rates of utilization of out-patient general health services. Borderline PD was significantly related to a poor marital relationship, a higher rate of physical disability, job difficulties, alcohol abuse, and psychosexual problems.

Although some believe there is a preponderance of females with borderline personality disorder, they do not always take into account prevalence of females in the populations studied.[19,20] Two studies did not find a higher female prevalence.[21,22]

Antisocial (Dissocial)

Antisocial is the most studied PD. Its prevalence has been assessed in large scale epidemiologic surveys, which employed standardized diagnostic criteria (Table 2).

In the ECA study, antisocial PD was investigated, and one month, six month, and lifetime prevalence rates of 0.5%, 1.2%, and 2.6% were found. There was a variation in the lifetime prevalence at three sites, ranging from 2.1% to 3.4%.[23] The lifetime prevalence rate for males was significantly higher (4.5%) than for females (0.8%), and the disorder was found predominantly in those under the age of 45, urban residents, and those who did not complete high school. The male excess occurred in every age and ethnic group. Among those with no disorder in the past year, the average duration of the disorder was 19 years. Typically it appeared at the age of eight, with a variety of problems at home and in

Table 2. Lifetime rates (%) of antisocial personality disorders (DSM-III) based on community surveys or relatives

Author and year of publication	Country	Sample size	Assessment method	Prevalence rate (%)
Baron et al., 1985 (14)	USA	376*	SIB, SADS	0.5*
		374**		0**
Bland et al., 1988a (26,27)	Canada	3258	DIS	3.7
Hwu et al., 1989 (28)	Taiwan	11,004	DIS	0.08
Kinzie et al., 1992 (29)	USA (Indian village)	131	SADS-L	0.4
Koegel et al., 1988 (32)	USA	328	DIS	20.8
Lee et al., 1990 (30)	Korea	3134 (urban)	DIS	2.1
		1966 (rural)		0.9
Maier et al., 1992 (10)	Germany	447	SCID	0.2
Reich et al., 1989b (15)	USA	235	PDQ	0.4
Robins et al., 1991 (23)	USA (ECA Program)	18,571	DIS	2.1–3.4***
Weissman & Myers, 1980 (17)	USA	511	SADS-L[†]	0.2
Wells et al., 1989 (25)	New Zealand	1498	DIS	3.1
Zimmerman & Coryell, 1990 (12)	USA	697	PDQ	0.9
			SIPD	3.0

[†] Current, not lifetime rates. * First-degree relatives of chronic schizophrenics, ** Normal control probands, *** Depending on the study site. Abbreviations: see Table 1.

school. Less than half of the diagnosed subjects had a significant record of arrest. Occupational problems were found in 94% of the sample, violence in 85%, and severe marital difficulties in 67%. Some form of substance abuse occurred in 84% of individuals with antisocial PD.[24] Associations with schizophrenia and mania were also found.

In the Christchurch Psychiatric Epidemiologic Study, carried out in New Zealand with a methodology similar to the ECA, six month and lifetime antisocial PD prevalence rates of 0.9% and 3.1% were found among a sample of 1498 adults, aged 18 to 64 years.[25] Males showed antisocial PD more frequently than females for both the six month (1.3% vs 0.5%) and lifetime (4.2% vs 0.5%) prevalence, but the differences did not achieve statistical significance. The authors also studied the one-year recovery rate, defined as the percentage of persons who had ever met criteria for a DIS DSM-III disorder but who had not experienced an episode or key symptoms of the disorder in the 12-months prior to the interview. The recovery rate for antisocial PD was 51.6%. However, it is possible that many recovered subjects were substance abusers, who no longer appeared personality disordered when abstinent.

In the Edmonton (Canada) study 3258 randomly selected adult household residents were interviewed with the DIS,[26,27] and 33.8% of the population met criteria for one or more disorders at some time in their life. A prevalence rate of 3.7% (6.5% for males and 0.8% for females) was found for antisocial PD. The disorder showed the highest rate in the age group 18–34, and among widowed, separated, and divorced subjects. The mean age of onset was 8 years for males and 9 years for females. All cases of antisocial personality had their onset before 20 years of age.

In Taiwan the rates of antisocial personality were considerably lower, ranging from 0.03% in rural villages to 1.4% in metropolitan Taipei.[28] This was consistent with the lower rates of most DSM-III disorders at the Taiwan site. In a survey of 131 subjects living in an Indian village in the western US, who were administered the SADS-L, only one male and no female cases were found.[29]

Lee et al.[30] performed a replication of the ECA study in the city of Seoul, Korea. They found a prevalence rate of antisocial personality disorder of 2.08% in a community sample of 3134. As in other studies there was a higher prevalence in males than females (3.54% vs 0.78%). Another replication of the ECA study[31] in Hong Kong, gave a prevalence of antisocial personality disorder of 2.78% in males and 0.53% in females in a sample of 7229 subjects. Antisocial personality disorder was one of the four most prevalent mental disorders found in males.

Both Reich et al.[15] and Zimmerman and Coryell,[12] using the PDQ, found considerably lower rates, 0.4% and 0.9% respectively. However, the rates increased to 3.0% when interviews were used, suggesting that self-reports may underestimate antisocial personality. Maier et al.,[10] however, using a structured interview, also found a low rate of 0.2% in Germany.

Interesting results were obtained by Koegel et al.[32] in a survey carried out among 328 homeless individuals living in the inner city of Los Angeles, who were administered the DIS, modified for use with a homeless population. An overall lifetime rate of 20.8% of antisocial PD was found compared to a rate of 4.7% in the Los Angeles sample in the ECA study (N = 3055). The risk ratio of having antisocial PD in the homeless as compared to the ECA sample was 4.4. The difference in rates was even more striking when the six month prevalence rate was considered. The rate among the homeless was 17.4% compared to 0.8% in the ECA sample, for a risk ratio of 21.8.

To summarize, antisocial PD seems to have a prevalence of around 3% in the general population, and to be more frequent among males than females, with sex ratios ranging from 2:1 to 7:1. It is also more common among younger adults, those living in urban areas, and the lower socioeconomic classes. People with a diagnosis of antisocial PD are also high users of medical services.

Avoidant

Reich et al.[15] and Baron et al.,[14] in their sample of relatives of normal probands, found no cases of avoidant personality (Table 1). Zimmerman and Coryell[12] reported rates ranging from 0.4% (PDQ) to 1.3% (SIPD). The rate reported by Maier et al.[10] (1.1%) was comparable to that obtained by Zimmerman and Coryell[12] and by Baron et al.[14] (1.6%) among relatives of schizophrenic probands.

Dependent

Reich et al.[15] and Zimmerman and Coryell,[12] using the PDQ, reported rates of 5.1% and 6.7% respectively (Table 1). However, the rates were lower when a structured interview was used (SIPD: 1.7%; SCID: 1.6%).[12,10]

Compulsive

The rates of compulsive disorder were comparable in two studies[12,15] in which the PDQ was used (6.4%[15] and 4.0%[12]). However, lower rates were reported with structured interviews, 1.7% with the SIPD[12] and 2.2% with the SCID.[10] Another study[33] carried out at the ECA Baltimore site, ascertained the prevalence of compulsive PD in the community, and found a prevalence of 1.7%. Males had a rate about five times higher than females. The disorder was also more frequent among white, highly educated, married, and employed subjects, and it was associated with anxiety disorders. However, the study derived the diagnosis from an interview originally not intended to diagnose PDs. This could mean that they identified adaptive obsessive-compulsive traits rather than a PD.

Passive-Aggressive

Using the PDQ, Zimmerman and Coryell[12] found a low rate (0.4%), while Reich et al,[15] in their study, which included only 235 subjects, found no cases. The rate was higher with an interview, suggesting that passive-aggressive persons may under-report on self-administered questionnaires.

Epidemiological studies carried out in psychiatric settings

Table 3 lists the main prevalence studies of PD carried out in in-patient and out-patient psychiatric samples.

To summarize, although the prevalence of PD among psychiatric out-patients and in-patients can be high, both in patients with only a PD and in those with an Axis I disorder (especially affective disorders), no final conclusion can be reached because the available studies reported very different prevalence rates. The differences are probably due to differences in sampling, diagnostic criteria, assessment methods, availability of mental health services, prevalence of Axis I disorders, and sociocultural factors. Even when authors use ICD or DSM criteria, they may have done so in different ways. There are, however, some consistencies across studies. The most prevalent PD seems to be borderline, both in in-patient and out-patient settings. The next most common PDs tend to be schizotypal and histrionic. These three disorders are also characterized by the lowest social functioning. They are especially common in in-patient settings, as their symptomatology often results in hospitalization due to suicidal behaviour, substance abuse, and cognitive-perceptual abnormalities. In out-patient settings, dependent and passive-aggressive PDs are also common.

In a study carried out among 2344 patients attending a public psychiatric facility and having a DSM-III diagnosis of PD, cluster B patients

Table 3. *Prevalence rates of personality disorders (PDs) among psychiatric patients*

Author and year of publication (Ref. no.)	Country	Sample size and setting	Classification system	Assessment instruments	% with PD	Remarks
Allan, 1991 (43)	UK	100 out-patients	RDC	Clinical interview	5	Alcohol abusers in treatment
Alnaes & Torgensen, 1988a (44,45)	Norway	298 out-patients	DSM-III	SIPD	81	97% had an Axis I diagnosis; about half had an affective disorder
Baer, *et al.*, 1990 (46)	USA	96 out-patients	DSM-III	SIPD	52	Obsessive-compulsive disorders. Dependent and histrionic PDs were the most common. Compulsive PD was found in only 6% of the sample.
Berger, 1985 (35)	Canada	486 out-patients	DSM-III	Clinical assessment	39	All patients seen in a private psychiatric practice over a period of five years
Castaneda & Franco, 1985 (47)	USA	1583 in-patients	DSM-III	Clinical assessment	6.4	Patients discharged from a psychiatric facility during one year; 101 received a primary diagnosis of PD
Charney *et al.*, 1981 (48)	USA	160 in-patients	DSM-III	Clinical assessment	61 / 14 / 23	64 unipolar nonmelancholic depressives 66 unipolar melancholic depressives 30 bipolar depressives
Cutting *et al.*, 1986 (49)	UK	100 in-patients	RDC	SAP	44	100 consecutive admissions with major psychiatric disorders. The proportion of patients with PD was comparable among different diagnostic groups (depressives 54%, schizophrenics 39%, manics 39%)
Dowson & Berrios, 1991 (50)	UK	74 in- and out-patients	DSM-III-R	PDQ-R	– / 4.5	Each patient had a mean number of PD diagnoses. Borderline (62%) and histrionic (61%) PDs were the most common.

Study	Sample	Classification	Assessment	%	Comments
Fabrega et al., 1991 (34) USA	18,179 out-patients	DSM-III	Initial Evaluation Form	12.9	Most frequent diagnoses were atypical, antisocial and borderline. Subjects with PD were males, 35 years or younger, socially impaired.
Friedman et al., 1983 (51) USA	53 in-patients	DSM-III	Clinical assessment	87	Depressed in-patients; 36 (78%) met criteria for borderline PD
Fyer et al., 1988 (52) USA	598 in-patients 501 in-patients	DSM-III	76 item checklist used to review medical records	54.1 54.3	Consecutive discharges from two psychiatric facilities. 23.2% and 19.8% of the two samples had borderline PD
Hyler & Lyons, 1988 (53) USA	358 (90% out-patients)	DSM-III	Specific assessment form	73.4	Patients in treatment with 287 US psychiatrists. The most common PD was borderline PD (21%), followed by compulsive PD (11%)
Jackson et al., 1991 (54) Australia	112	DSM-III-R	SIPD	67	21% had one PD, 46% had >2 PDs. Schizophrenia associated with antisocial and schizotypal PDs
Kass et al., 1985 (22) USA	609 out-patients	DSM-III	4-point rating format	51	Borderline was the most frequent PD (11%)
Kastrup, 1987 (55) Denmark	11.340 (in-patients)	ICD-8	Clinical assessment	18.3(a) 16.7(a) 15.2(b) 15.7(b)	a=revolving door patients, first diagnosis and last diagnosis b=non revolving door patients, first diagnosis and last diagnosis
Kennedy et al., 1990 (56) Canada	44 (in-patients)	DSM-III-R	MGMI BSI	93	Patients with eating disorders. Borderline, dependent and passive-aggressive PDs were the most common
Kroll et al., 1981 (57) USA	117 (in-patients)	DSM-III	DIB	18	Assessment focused on borderline PD
Loranger, 1990 (38) USA	5143 (a)	DSM-II (a)	Clinical assessment	19.1	Diagnoses made according to the DSM-II in the years 1975-79
	5771 (b) (in-patients)	DSM-III (b)		49.2	Diagnoses made according to the DSM-III in the years 1981-85

Table 3. (*contd.*)

Author and year of publication (Ref. no.)	Country	Sample size and setting	Classification system	Assessment instruments	% with PD	Remarks
Loranger et al., 1991 (58)	USA	84 (in-patients)	DSM-III	PDE	58.3(a) 50(b)	Patients evaluated at entry (a) and at follow-up (b). Borderline, avoidant, dependent and masochistic PDs were the most common
McGlashan, 1986 (59)	USA	532 (in-patients)	DSM-III	Clinical assessment	32	Patients who met DSM-III criteria or Gunderson's criteria for borderline PD
Mezzich et al., 1982 (60)	USA	1111 (in- and out-patients)	DSM-III & ICD-9	Initial Evaluation Form	21.4	For 33 (3%) patients an Axis II diagnosis was primary
Mezzich et al., 1990 (61)	USA	4,141 (38% in-patients, 62% out-patients)	DSM-III & ICD-9	Initial Evaluation Form	14.0	PD first cluster=7%; PD second cluster=45%; PD third cluster=19%; PD fourth cluster=30%. Most frequent Axis I diagnoses: somatoform disorders (36%) and substance abuse (25%)
Nace et al.,1991 (62)	USA	100 (in-patients)	DSM-III-R	SCID-II	57	100 middle-class in-patient substance abusers
Numberg et al., 1991 (63)	USA	110 (out-patients)	DSM-III-R	Semistructured assessment	62	Patients with any minor axis I diagnosis. Avoidant (24%), borderline (20%) and histrionic (17%) were the most common PD
Nussbaum & Rogers, 1992 (64)	Canada	82 (in-patients)	DSM-III-R	SCID-PQ	–	The SCID-PQ yielded very few false negatives and moderate false positives.
Oldham et al., 1992 (65)	USA	100 (in-patients)	DSM-III-R	SCID-II	–	Patients assigned 290 PD diagnoses. Borderline, avoidant and dependent PDs most common.
Oldham & Skodol, 1991 (66)	USA	129,268 (in- and out-patients)	DSM-III & ICD-9	Clinical assessment	10.8	All patients served by the New York State Office of Mental Health in one year. Of

Study	Country	Criteria	Instrument	%	Comments
Pfohl et al., 1986 (67)	USA	DSM-III	SIPD	51	all PD patients, 17.2% had a diagnosis of borderline PD. Schizoaffective disorders, major affective disorders, dysthymia, substance abuse were more common among PD patients. Histrionic (30%) and borderline (29%) most common. 54% of the PD had two or more PDs
Pilgrim & Mann, 1990 (68)	UK	ICD-10	SAP	36	First admissions in one year. Anxious and impulsive PDs most common.
Pilkonis & Frank, 1988 (69)	USA	DSM-III	Hirschfeld-Klerman Personality Battery, PAS	48	Patients with recurrent unipolar depression. Most common PDs were avoidant (30.4%) and compulsive (18.6%)
Reich, 1987 (21)	USA	DSM-III	SIPD PDQ MCMI	48.8 60.0 66.7	45% had a consensus diagnosis of PD. More women with histrionic PD and more men with paranoid, compulsive and antisocial PDs
Reich & Troughton, 1988 (13)	USA	DSM-III	SIDP SIPD PDQ	43 55 20	Panic patients assessed with the SIPD. Out-patients assessed with the SIDP. Normal controls assessed with the PDQ
Ross et al., 1988 (70)	Canada	DSM-III	DIS	47	501 addicts. 47% had a diagnosis of anti-social PD
Rounsaville et al., 1991 (71)	USA	DSM-III-R	SADS	7.7	Cocaine abusers. 7.7% had a diagnosis of antisocial PD
Shea et al., 1990 (72)	USA	DSM-III	PAF	74	Major depressives in the NIMH Treatment of Depression Collaborative Research Program. 57% of those with PD had a diagnosis of two or more PDs. Compulsive, avoidant, dependent and paranoid most frequent diagnoses.

Sample sizes: 131 (in-patients); 120 (in-patients); 119 (out-patients); 170 (out-patients); 88(a), 82(b), 40(a); 501 (out-patients); 298 (in- and out-patients); 239 (out-patients).

Table 3. (contd.)

Author and year of publication (Ref. no.)	Country	Sample size and setting	Classification system	Assessment instruments	% with PD	Remarks
Turner et al., 1991 (73)	USA	68 (out-patients)	DSM-III-R	SCID-II	37	Patients with social phobia. Over 75% received subthreshold ratings for one or more PDs. Avoidant and obsessive PD most common.
Tyrer et al., 1983 (74)	UK	316 (all out-patients except 12 pts)	ICD-8	PAS	39.9	All patients had a diagnosis of neurosis. Anankastic personality disorder was the most common
Zanarini et al., 1987 (75)	USA	43 (in-patients)	DSM-III	DIDP	81	97% of the PDs had two or more PDs. Borderline PD was most frequent (26%)
Zimmerman et al., 1988 (76)	USA	66 (in-patients)	DSM-III	SIDP	57.6 36.4	Based on patient interview Based on informant interview

Abbreviations: RDC, Research Diagnostic Criteria; DSM, Diagnostic and Statistical Manual of Mental Disorders; ICD, International Statistical Classification of Diseases Related Health Problems; SIPD, Structured Interview for Personality Disorders; SAP, Standardized Assessment of Personality; PDQ, Personality Diagnostic Questionnaire; MGMI, Million Clinical Multiaxial Inventory; BSI, Borderline Syndrome Index; DIB, Diagnostic Interview for Borderlines; SCID, Structured Clinical Interviews for DSM; PDE, Personality Disorder Examination; PAS, Personality Assessment Schedule; DIS, Diagnostic Interview Schedule; PAF, Personality Assessment Form; DIDP, Diagnostic Interview for Personality Disorders.

were the most frequent and cluster A patients the least.[34] There was highly significant demographic variation manifest across PD clusters. In the only study which investigated PD rates among those seen in a private psychiatric practice (N = 486), they were diagnosed in 39% of the patients seen.[35] Borderline (9.7%) and obsessive-compulsive (8.2%) were the most frequently observed.

Some studies have compared the hospital admission rates for PD over time, and they allow us to assess the impact of diagnostic changes. Mors[36] has shown that in Denmark sex- and age-standardized rates of first-admitted borderlines significantly increased during the 16-year interval 1970–85. There was no sex difference, but the age group 15–34 especially contributed to the increase, which was particularly remarkable in urban areas, and might be explained in terms of a change in diagnostic habits. This hypothesis received support from another analysis of Danish admissions to psychiatric institutions in the years 1975, 1980, and 1985. In those years the increase in borderline diagnosis (5% to 20%) in men paralleled a decrease in the diagnosis of psychopathy (22% to 7%).[37] The authors suggest that those previously diagnosed as psychopathic deviants were subsequently labelled borderlines. The shift in diagnosis was less marked for females.

This same phenomenon, i.e., a change in diagnostic practice has been studied at one of the largest university-affiliated psychiatric hospitals in the USA.[38] Comparing the diagnoses given to hospitalized patients in the last five years of the DSM-II era (N = 5143) with those given in the first five years of the DSM-III era (N = 5771), a marked increase was found in the diagnosis of PD, together with a decrease in the diagnosis of schizophrenia, and a corresponding increase in the diagnosis of affective disorders. The percentage of patients with a diagnosis of PD (19.1% to 49.2%) increased more than twofold. The most frequent diagnostic categories employed since the introduction of the DSM-III were atypical/mixed/other PD (33%) and borderline (27%). Another study assessed the proportion of patients with PD among all hospitalized cases of non-psychotic mental disorders in military personnel in the US Navy from 1981–1984.[39] The overall sample included 27,210 cases. Among them, 4581 (16.8%) had a PD as the primary diagnosis. In New Zealand a survey was made of all patients admitted to psychiatric hospitals over a seven year period with an ICD-9 primary diagnosis of personality disorders (N = 6447).[40] Despite a decrease in the total number of admissions, the relative totals for each personality disorder remained consistent. The most common diagnosis was an unspecified

PD, and it accounted for 45% of the total sample. The next most common was asthenic PD.

In the US on a selected day in 1986, there were a total of 3893 persons under care in some in-patient psychiatric facility, with a primary diagnosis of PD. This corresponded to 2.4% of the total number of in-patients on that date.[41] In the same year there were 29,910 admissions with a primary diagnosis of PD, 1.9% of all admissions. The median length of hospital stay for in-patients with a diagnosis of PD was nine days. Among all those under out-patient care on the same day, there were 81,731 or 5.9% of the total, with a diagnosis of PD. In the same year 136,903 people or 6.4% were admitted to out-patient care with a PD diagnosis.

The epidemiological findings in treated samples are especially important if we bear in mind that the presence of a PD among those suffering from other mental disorders can be a major predictor of the natural history and treatment outcome.[6]

Conclusions

The epidemiology of PDs has not received the same amount of attention as that of many other psychiatric disorders. In the last few years the situation has changed, and we now have data on the prevalence of PD in the community and in psychiatric facilities. Community data come primarily from three studies[10-12] with a total sample of about 1300 subjects from two countries, Germany and the US. There are excellent national and cross-national epidemiological data on antisocial personality disorder, based on the same diagnostic methods. There are almost no data on other PDs from countries other than Germany and the US. The lack of studies from developing countries is especially noteworthy because the role of sociocultural factors has yet to be determined.

One important methodological problem is that some PDs have a very low prevalence rate. Consequently, epidemiological surveys carried out among the general population may require very large samples in order to identify a sufficient number of cases to study demographic correlates and the association of PD with other psychiatric disorders.

Many of the PDs are at an early stage of construct validation. Further research should probably follow the general recommendations for validating a psychiatric disorder. These include the need to delineate a proposed disorder from other disorders. Given the overlap of the PDs, this will be a challenging task. Another criterion is external validation, and there are a number of psychological tests and behavioural indicators that might be used to establish construct validity. Biological markers will also be important in future research as another source of external validation.

Another method of validation is to determine whether the course or natural history of PDs justifies their differentiation. Few such studies have been done, because of the time and cost of prospective designs, but longitudinal studies can provide information not available from cross-sectional ones. They could identify predictors of future PDs, modifying variables, and medical and social service needs. They also offer an opportunity to examine the effect of temperament as an important pre-disposing variable. Another issue that could be explored in this way is the temporal stability of PDs. Although as defined in the ICD-10 and DSM-III, PDs are long-lasting disorders, very limited data are available regarding this. For this reason it would be worth investigating the epidemiology of PDs in different age groups, as an indication of the course of PDs. Longitudinal studies will also provide evidence for the validity of the concept of PD as constant maladaptive behaviour across time and environmental circumstances.[42]

Finally, treatment response is also a validator. Although PDs are considered stable and long lasting, it is possible that effective treatments will ultimately be developed, as with other psychiatric disorders, and treatment response could also be used to validate the different types of PD. There has been a remarkable advance in our understanding of the epidemiology of PDs in the last few years. As this continues, we should better understand not only the PDs, but also other mental disorders.

References

1   Casey, P.R. Epidemiology of personality disorders. In Tyrer, P. (ed.) *Personality Disorders: Diagnosis, Management and Course*. London: Wright, 1988.

2   Merikangas, K.R. & Weissman, M.M. Epidemiology of DSM-III Axis II personality disorders. In: Frances, A.J. & Hales, R.E. (eds), *APA Annual Review*, vol. 5, *Psychiatry Update*, pp. 258–78. Washington, DC: American Psychiatric Press, 1986.

3   Merikangas, K.R. Epidemiology of DSM-III personality disorders. In Michels, R. *et al.*, (eds.). *Psychiatry*, vol 3, pp 1–16. Philadelphia: Lippincott, 1989.

4   Weissman, M.M. The epidemiology of personality disorders: A 1990 update. *Journal of Personality Disorders*, 1993; **7**, 44–62.

5   Andreoli, A., Gressot, G., Aapro, N., Tricot, L. & Gognalons, M.Y. Personality disorders as a predictor of outcome. *Journal of Personality Disorders*, 1989; **3**: 307–20.

6   Reich, J.H. & Green, A.I. Effect of personality disorders on outcome of treatment. *Journal of Nervous and Mental Disease*, 1991; **179**: 74–82.

7   Neugebauer, R., Dohrenwend, B.P. & Dohrenwend, B.S. Formulation of hypotheses about the true prevalence of functional psychiatric disorders among adults in the US. In Dohrenwend, B.P., Dohrenwend, B.S., Gould, M.S., Link, B., Neugebauer, R. & Wunsch-Hitzir, R. (eds.). *Mental Illness in the United States: Epidemiological Estimates*, pp. 56–92. New York: Praeger, 1980.

8   Perry, C. & Vaillant, G.E. Personality Disorders. In Kaghan, H.I., Sadock, B.J. (eds.). *Comprehensive Textbook of Psychiatry*, pp. 1352–86. Baltimore: William & Wirekins, 1989.

9   Casey, P.R. & Tyrer, P.J. Personality, functioning and symptomatology. *Journal of Psychiatric Research*, 1986; **20**: 363–74.

10 Maier, W., Lichtermann, D., Klingler, T. & Heun, R. Prevalences of personality disorders (DSM-III-R) in the community. *Journal of Personality Disorders*, 1992; **6**: 187–96.

11 Reich, J., Boerstler, H., Yates, W. & Nduaguba, M. Utilization of medical resources in persons with DSM-III personality disorders in a community sample. *International Journal of Psychiatry in Medicine*, 1989a; **19**: 1–9.

12 Zimmerman, M. & Coryell, W.H. Diagnosing personality disorders in the community. *Archives of General Psychiatry*, 1990; **47**: 527–31.

13 Reich, J. & Troughton, E. Frequency of DSM-III personality disorders in patients with panic disorder: comparison with psychiatric and normal control subjects. *Psychiatry Research*, 1988; **26**: 89–100.

14 Baron, M., Gruen, R., Rainer, J.D., Kane, J., Asnis, L. & Lord, S. A family study of schizophrenic and normal control probands: Implications for the spectrum concept of schizophrenia. *American Journal of Psychiatry*, 1985; **142**: 447–55.

15 Reich, J.H., Yates, W. & Nduaguba, M. Prevalence of DSM-III personality disorders in the community. *Social Psychiatry*, 1989b; **24**: 12-16.

16 Nestadt, G., Romanoski, AJ., Chahal, R., Merchant, A., Folstein, M.F., Gruenberg, E.M., & McHugh, P.R. An epidemiological study of histrionic personality disorder. *Psychological Medcine*, 1990; **20**: 413–22.

17 Weissman, M.M. & Myers, J.K. Psychiatric disorders in a US community. *Acta Psychiatrica Scandinavica*, 1980; **62**: 99–111.

18 Swartz, M., Blazer, D., George, L. & Winfield, I. Estimating the prevalence of borderline personality disorder in the community. *Journal of Personality Disorders*, 1990; **4**: 257–72.

19 Akhtar, S., Byrne, J.P. & Doghramji, K. The demographic profile of borderline personality disorder. *Journal of Clinical Psychiatry*, 1986; **47**:196-198.

20 Widiger, T.A. & Weissman, M.M. Epidemiology of borderline personality disorder. *Hospital and Community Psychiatry*, 1991; **42**: 1015–21.

21 Reich, J. Sex distribution of DSM-III personality disorders in psychiatric outpatients. *American Journal of Psychiatry*, 1987; **144**: 485–8.

22 Kass, F., Skodol, A.E., Charles, E., Spitzer, R.L. & Williams, J.B.W. Scaled ratings of DSM-III personality disorders. *American Journal of Psychiatry*, 1985; **142**: 627–30.

23   Robins, L., Tipp, J. & Przybeck, T. Antisocial personality. In Robins, L. & Regier, D.A. (eds.). *Psychiatric Disorders in America. The ECA Study*, pp. 258–90. New York: Free Press, 1991.

24   Regier, D.A., Farmer, M.E., Rae, D.S., Locke, B.Z., Keith, S.J., Judd, L.L. & Goodwin, F.K. Comorbidity of mental disorders with alcohol and other drug abuse. *JAMA*, 1990; **264**: 2511–18.

25   Wells, E.J., Bushnell, J.A., Hornblow, A.R., Joyce, P.R. & Oakley-Browne, M.A. Christchurch psychiatric epidemiology study. Part I: Methodology and lifetime prevalence for specific psychiatric disorders. *Australian and New Zealand Journal of Psychiatry*, 1989; **23**: 315–26

26   Bland, R.C., Newman, S.C. & Orn, H. Age of onset of psychiatric disorders. *Acta Psychiatrica Scandinavica*, 1988a; **77** (Suppl 338): 43–9.

27   Bland, R.C., Orn. H. & Newman, S.C. Lifetime prevalence of psychiatric disorders in Edmonton. *Acta Psychiatrica Scandinavica*, 1988b; **77** (Suppl 338): 24–32

28   Hwu, H.G., Yeh, E.K. & Chang, L.Y. Prevalence of psychiatric disorders in Taiwan defined by the Chinese Diagnostic Interview Schedule. *Acta Psychiatrica Scandinavica*, 1989; **79**: 136–47.

29   Kinzie, J.D., Leung, P.K., Boehnlein, J., Matsunaga, D., Johnson, R., Manson, S., Shore, J.H., Heinz, J. & Williams, M. Psychiatric epidemiology of an Indian village: A 19-year replication study. *Journal of Nervous and Mental Disease*, 1992; **180**: 33–9.

30   Lee, C.K., Kwak, Y.S., Yamamoto, J., Rhee, H., Kim, Y.S., Han, J.H., Choi, J.O. & Lee, Y.H. Psychiatric Epidemiology in Korea, Part I: Gender and Age Differences in Seoul. *Journal of Nervous and Mental Disease*, 1990; **178**: 242–52.

31   Chen, C., Wong, J., Lee, N., Chan-Ho, M., Lau, J.T. & Fung, M. The Shatin community mental health survey in Hong Kong. II. Major findings. *Archives of General Psychiatry*, 1993; **50**, 125–33.

32   Koegel, P., Burnam, M.A., & Farr, R.K. The prevalence of specific psychiatric disorders among homeless individuals in the inner city of Los Angeles. *Archives of General Psychiatry*, 1988; **45**: 1085–92.

33   Nestadt, G., Romanoski, A.J., Brown, C.H., Chahal, R., Merchant, A., Folstein, M.F., Gruenberg, E.M. & McHugh, P.R. DSM-III compulsive personality disorder: An epidemiological survey. *Psychological Medicine*, 1991; **21**: 461–71.

34   Fabrega, H., Ulrich, R., Pilkonis, P. & Mezzich, J. On the homogenity of personality disorder clusters. *Comprehensive Psychiatry*, 1991; **32**: 373–85.

35   Berger, J. Private practice: The first five years. *Canadian Journal of Psychiatry*, 1985; **30**: 566–71.

36   Mors, O. Increasing incidence of borderline states in Denmark from 1970-1985. *Acta Psychiatrica Scandinavica*, 1988; **77**: 575–83.

37   Simonsen, E. & Mellergard, M. Trends in the use of the borderline diagnosis in Denmark from 1975 to 1985. *Journal of Personality Disorders*, 1988; **2**: 102–8.

38   Loranger, A.W. The impact of DSM-III on diagnostic practice in a University Hospital. *Archives of General Psychiatry*, 1990; **47**: 672–5.

39   Kilbourne, B., Goodman, J. & Hilton, S. Predicting personality disorder diagnoses of hospitalized navy personnel. *Military Medicine*, 1991; **156**: 354–7.

40   Mulder, R.T. Personality disorders in New Zealand hospitals. *Acta Psychiatrica Scandinavica*, 1991; **84**: 197–202.

41   NIMH. *Mental Health, United States, 1990*. Manderscheid, R.W. & Sonnenschein, M.A. (eds.). DHHS Pub. No. (ADM) 90–1708. Washington: Superintendent of Documents, U.S., Government Printing Office, 1990.

42   Rutter, M. Temperament, personality and personality disorder. *British Journal of Psychiatry*, 1987; **150**: 443–58.

43   Allan, C.A. Psychological symptoms, psychiatric disorder and alcohol dependence amongst men and women attending a community-based voluntary agency and an Alcohol Treatment Unit. *British Journal of Addiction*, 1991; **86**: 419–27.

44   Alnaes, R. & Torgersen, S. The relationship between DSM-III symptom disorders (Axis I) and personality disorders (Axis II) in an outpatient population. *Acta Psychiatrica Scandinavica*, 1988a; **78**: 485–92.

45   Alnaes, R. & Torgersen, S. DSM-III symptom disorders (Axis I) and personality disorders (Axis II) in an Outpatient Population. *Acta Psychiatrica Scandinavica*, 1988b; **78**: 348–55.

46   Baer, L., Jenike, M.A., Ricciardi, J.N., Holland, A.D., Seymour, R.J., Minichiello, W.E. & Buttolph, L. Standardized assessment of personality disorders in obsessive-compulsive disorder. *Archives of General Psychiatry*, 1990; **47**: 826.

47   Castenada, R. & Franco, H. Sex and ethnic distribution of borderline personality disdorder in an inpatient sample. *American Journal of Psychiatry*, 1985; **142**: 1202–3.

48   Charney, D.S., Nelson, J.C. & Quinlan, D.M. Personality traits and disorder in depression. *American Journal of Psychiatry*, 1981; **138**: 1601–4.

49   Cutting, J., Cowen, P.J., Mann, A.H. & Jenkins, R. Personality and psychosis: use of the standardized assessment of personality, *Acta Psychiatrica Scandinavica*, 1986; **73**: 87–92.

50   Dowson, J.H. & Berrios, G.E. Factor strucure of DSM-III-R personality disorders shown by self-report questionnaire: implications for classifying and assessing personality disorders. *Acta Psychiatrica Scandinavica*, 1991; **84**: 555–60.

51   Friedman, R.C., Aronoff, M.S., Clarkin, J.F., Corn, R. & Hurt, S.W. History of suicidal behaviour in depressed borderline inpatients. *America Journal of Psychiatry*, 1983; **140**: 1023–6.

52   Fyer, M.R., Frances, A.J., Sulivan, T., Hurt, S.W., Clarkin, J. Comorbidity of borderline personality disorder. *Archives of General Psychiatry*, 1988; **45**: 348–52.

53   Hyler, S.E. &Lyons, M. Factor analysis of the DSM-III personality disorder clusters: a replication. *Comprehensive Psychiatry*, 1988; **29**: 304–8.

54   Jackson, H.J., Whiteside, H.L., Bates, G.W., Bell, R., Rudd, R.P. & Edwards, J. Diagnosing personality disorders in psychiatric inpatients. *Acta Psychiatrica Scandinavica*, 1991; **83**: 206–13.

55   Kastrup, M. Who became revolving door patients? Findings from a nation-wide cohort of first time admitted psychiatric patients. *Acta Psychiatrica Scandinavica*, 1987; **76**: 80–8.

56   Kennedy, S.H., McVey, G. & Katz, R. Personality disorders in anorexia nervosa and bulimia nervosa. *Journal of Psychiatry, Res.*, 1990; **24**: 259–9.

57. Kroll, J., Sines L., Martin, K., Lari, S., Pyle, R. & Zander, J. Borderline personality disorder: construct validity of the concept. *Archives of General Psychiatry*, 1981; **38**: 1021–6.

58   Loranger, A.W., Lenzenweger, M.F., Gartner, A.F., Susman, V.L., Herzig, J., Zammit, G.K., Gartner, J.D., Abrams, R.C. & Young, R.C. Trait-state artifacts and the diagnosis of personality disorders. *Archives of General Psychiatry*, 1991; 48: 720–8.

59   McGlashan, T.H. The Chestnut Lodge Follow-up Study III. Long-term outcome of borderline personalities. *Archives of General Psychiatry*, 1986; 43: 20–30.

60   Mezzich, J.E., Coffman, G.A. & Goodpastor, S.M. A format for DSM-III diagnostic formulation: experience with 1,111 consecutive patients. *American Journal of Psychiatry*, 1982; **139**: 591–6.

61   Mezzich, J.E., Ahn, C.W., Fabrega, H. & Pilkonis, P.A. Patterns of psychiatric comorbidity in a large population presenting for care. In Maser JD, Cloninger CR, eds. *Comorbidity of Mood and Anxiety Disorders*, pp. 189–204. Washington: American Psychiatric Press, 1990.

62   Nace, E.P., Davis, C.W. & Gaspari, J. Axis II Comorbidity in substance abusers. *American Journal of Psychiatry*, 1991; **148**: 118–20.

63   Nurnberg, G.H., Raskin, M., Levine, P.E., Pollack, S., Siegel, O. & Prince, R. The comorbidity of borderline personality disorder and other DSM-III-R Axis II personality disorders. *American Journal of Psychiatry*, 1991; **148**: 1371–7.

64   Nussbaum, D. & Rogers, R. Screening psychiatric patients for Axis II disorders. *Canadian Journal of Psychiatry*, 1992; **37**: 658–60.

65   Oldham, J.M. & Skodol, A.E. Personality disorders in the public sector. *Hospital and Community Psychiatry*, 1991; **42**: 481–7.

66   Oldham, J.M., Skodol, A.E., Kellman, H.D., Hyler, S.E., Rosnick, L. & Davies, M. Diagnosis of DSM-III personality disorders by two structured interviews: patterns of comorbidity. *American Journal of Psychiatry*, 1992; **142**: 213–20.

67   Pfohl, B., Coryell, W., Zimmerman, M. & Stangl D. DSM-III personality disorders: Diagnostic overlap and inter consistency of individual DSM-III criteria. *Comprehensive Psychiatry*, 1986; **27**: 21–34.

68   Pilgrim, J. & Mann, A. Use of the ICD-10 version of the standardized assessment of personality to determine the prevalence of personality disorder in psychiatric in-patients. *Psychological Medicine*, 1990; **20**: 985–92.

69   Pilkomis, P.A. & Frank, E. Personality pathology in recurrent depression: nature, prevalence, and relationship to treatment response. *American Journal of Psychiatry*, 1988; **145**: 435–41.

70   Ross, H.E., Glaser, F.B. & Germanson, T. The prevalence of psychiatric disorders in patients with alcohol and other drug problems. *Archives of Genergl Psychiatry*, 1988; **45**: 1023.

71   Rounsaville, B.J., Anton, S.F., Carroll, K., Budde, D., Prusoff, B.A. & Gawin, F. Psychiatric diagnoses of treatment-seeking cocaine abusers. *Archives of General Psychiatry*, 1991; **48**: 43.

72   Shea, M.T., Pilkonis, P.A., Beckham, E. Collins, J.F., Elkins, I., Sorsky, S.M. & Docherty, J.P. Personality disorders and treatment outcome in the NIMH Treatment of Depression Collaborative Research Program. *American Journal of Psychiatry*, 1990; **147**: 711–17.

73   Turner, S.S., Beidel, D.C., Borden, J.W., Stanley, M.A. & Jacob, R.G. Social Phobia: Axis I and II correlates. *Journal of Abnormal Psychology*, 1991; **100**: 102–6.

74   Tyrer, P., Casey, P. & Gall, J. Relationship between neurosis and personality disoder. *British Journal of Psychiatry*, 1983; **142**: 404–8.

75   Zanarini, M.C., Frankenburg, F.R., Chauncey, D.L. & Gunderson, J.G. The diagnostic interview for personality disorders: Interrater and test-retest reliability. *Comprehensive Psychiatry*, 1987; **28**: 467–80.

76   Zimmerman, M., Pfohl, B., Coryell, W., Stangl, D. & Coranthal, J.L.C. Diagnosing personality disorder in depressed patients. A comparison of patient informant interviews. *Archives of General Psychiatry*, 1988; **45**: 733–7.

International personality disorder examination (IPDE)

Armand W. Loranger

Background and History

One of the aims of the World Health Organization (WHO) and US Alcohol, Drug Abuse and Mental Health Administration (ADAMHA) joint program on psychiatric diagnosis and classification was the development and standardization of diagnostic assessment instruments for use in clinical research around the world.[1] The International Personality Disorder Examination (IPDE) is a semistructured clinical interview originally designed to assess the personality disorders (PDs) in the ICD-10[2] and DSM-III-R[3] classification systems, and subsequently modified for compatibility with DSM-IV.[4]

The IPDE is an outgrowth and adaptation for international use of the Personality Disorder Examination (PDE) (Loranger, 1988).[5] To facilitate the development of the IPDE, beginning in 1985 several international workshops were convened. At these meetings WHO and ADAMHA officials, together with representatives of the international psychiatric community, discussed the format of the interview, the wording of items, and the development of a scoring manual. Frequent revisions were made to reflect the experience of interviewers with trial versions. Investigators at the various centres involved in the field trial described in this volume translated the instrument into the following languages: Dutch, French, German, Hindi, Japanese, Kannada, Norwegian, Swahili, and Tamil. The translations were back-translated into English by a psychiatrist or psychologist who had not seen the original English version. Variations and problems in the back-translation were then reviewed with those who undertook the original translation, and corrections were made when indicated. Later, translations were made into other languages, including Danish, Italian, Spanish, Russian, and Estonian. Additional translations are contemplated.

Particular problems arise when the interview is used with subjects who are illiterate and speak a regional or tribal dialect. Since written and spoken language are quite different in such populations, the interviewer must frequently depart from the literal text and improvise an equivalent question on the spot, in order to maintain communication with the subject. Although this is a potential source of error variance, the examiner's familiarity with the scope and meaning of the diagnostic criteria and with the intent of the original IPDE question, should keep such error within tolerable limits.

Structure of the IPDE

The IPDE is arranged in a format that attempts to provide the optimal balance between a spontaneous, natural clinical interview and the requirements of standardization and objectivity. At the beginning of the interview the subject is given the following instructions: 'The questions I am going to ask concern what you are like most of the time. I'm interested in what has been typical of you throughout your life, and not just recently. If you have changed and your answers might have been different at some time in the past, be sure to let me know.'

The questions flow in a natural sequence that is congenial to the clinician. They are arranged under six headings: work, self, interpersonal relationships, affects, reality testing, and impulse control. The headings are not only convenient labels, but they play an organizational or thematic role. At times the overlapping nature of the six domains required a somewhat arbitrary allocation of questions. For efficiency and convenience sometimes a question extends beyond the scope of the section where it appears. For example, many obsessive-compulsive criteria are best assessed in the context of work functioning, but behaviour outside the realm of work is also considered, even though the questions appear in the 'work' section of the interview.

The sections are usually introduced by open-ended inquiries that offer the subject an opportunity to discuss the topic as much as he chooses. This helps to develop a set for the questions that follow, and provides a transition from the focus of the previous section. Although they are not scored as such, these introductory remarks of the subject provide a background against which to judge the clinical significance of some of the replies to the specific questions that follow. At times the comments also facilitate the task of the examiner in deciding whether to probe or pursue certain aspects of the subject's responses.

The criterion and its number, together with the name of the disorder, appear above the questions designed to assess it. Since the questions are merely an attempt to get at the criterion, this serves to remind the examiner what he is actually rating. When there is no major difference between an ICD and DSM criterion, they are assessed together by identical questions. This occurs as often as possible to prevent the combined ICD-DSM version of the interview from becoming too long or unwieldy. Some criteria are followed by the designation *partial*, an indication that the item does not assess the entire criterion. This is done to preserve the topical focus of the interview. For example, it is more appropriate to inquire about an identity disorder in the sexual realm, when the subject of sex is being discussed, than to attempt to cover other manifestations of an identity disorder, such as uncertainty about values or career choice, at the same point in the interview.

There appears to be no consensus about how long a behaviour should be present before it can be considered a personality trait. The IPDE has adopted the conservative convention that it should exist for a span of at least five years. Consideration was given to a three-year requirement, but it was decided that might too frequently lead to confounding episodic mental illnesses or responses to unusual or special life situations with the more enduring behaviour associated with personality. Some may feel this is too exacting, especially when applied to adolescents. Since users of the IPDE will differ in their predilection for making PD diagnoses in adolescents, those who prefer a three-year requirement may adopt it for that age group. They should specify, however, that they have departed from the standard instructions. The use of anything less than a five-year timeframe with subjects over 20 years of age is discouraged.

ICD-10, DSM-III-R, and DSM-IV date the onset of the first manifestations of a PD to childhood, adolescence, or early adulthood. For that reason the IPDE takes the somewhat arbitrary position, that the requirements for at least one criterion of a disorder must have been fulfilled prior to age 25, before that particular disorder can be diagnosed. Age 25 years rather than an earlier age was selected to allow more informed and accurate judgments about many of the adult-oriented PD criteria. Clinical tradition notwithstanding, it is possible that personality transformations may occur in midlife or old age, and that a true PD may emerge *de novo* at that time. In the absence of empirical data, rather than encourage premature closure on the subject, there is provision in the IPDE for an optional *late onset* diagnosis. The interview also provides the option of making a *past* diagnosis in someone who previously met the requirements, but does not evidence the behaviour currently (past 12 months).

Administration and scoring

Much of the behaviour described in the criteria of ICD-10, DSM-III-R, and DSM-IV exists on a continuum with normality. The IPDE scoring is based on the convention that a behaviour or trait may be absent or normal (0), exaggerated or accentuated (1), and criterion level or pathological (2). A few criteria are not applicable to certain subjects, and are scored 'NA'. A '?' scoring category is reserved for those rare occasions when a subject, despite encouragement, refuses to answer a question or states that he/she is unable to do so. It is not used to designate uncertainty on the part of the examiner about rating the item.

No single formula was used in developing the guidelines in the scoring manual. They are based on interpretations of the criteria by the author of the instrument, and were revised after discussions with the clinicians who participated in the field trial. Clinical judgement, common sense, and practical experience with the interview shaped the final version of the guidelines. The boxed text contains a sample item from the IPDE demonstrating the format, type of questions, and scoring guidelines.

Initial replies of the subject that suggest a positive reply are rarely sufficient for scoring a criterion. They must be supplemented and supported by convincing descriptions or examples. The examiner uses clinical judgement to determine the length of the descriptions and the number of examples. Although there is a standard set of probes, they must be augmented by an adequate clinical examination of the subject.

The interviewer scores the IPDE item-by-item, as he progresses through the interview. The scores are combined for diagnostic purposes at the conclusion of the interview. Although this may be done clerically using a set of step-by-step algorithmic directions, the most efficient method is to use a program especially designed for personal computers. It is written with operator prompts, and the user responds to questions regarding the task to be performed and the management of the data, which may be sent to a printer and saved in a disk file. The entire procedure takes 5 to 10 minutes.

Scope of the IPDE

The IPDE is not designed to survey the entire realm of personality. Its purpose is to identify those traits and behaviours that are relevant to an assessment of the criteria for personality disorders in the ICD-10 and DSM-IV classification systems. It neglects many neutral, positive, and

Sample of IPDE item

The questions I am going to ask concern what you are like most of the time. I'm interested in what has been typical of you throughout your life, and not just recently. If you have changed and your answers might have been different at some time in the past, be sure to let me know.

I. WORK

If the subject has rarely or never worked, and is not a housewife (homemaker), student, or recent graduate, circle NA for 1 and proceed to 2.

I would like to begin by discussing your life at work (school). How well do you usually function in your work (at school)?

What annoyances or problems keep occurring in your work (at school)?

---

1.   0   1   2   ?   0   1   2   ?   NA
            Is excessively devoted to work and productivity to the exclusion of leisure activities and friendships (not accounted for by obvious economic necessity)
            Obsessive Compulsive: 3

Do you spend so much time working that you don't have any time left for anything else?
  If yes: Tell me about it.

Do you spend so much time working that you (also) neglect other people?
  If yes: Tell me about it.

The examiner should be alert to the use of rationalizations to defend the behaviour. The fact that work itself may be pleasurable to the subject should not influence the scoring. There is no requirement that the subject actually enjoy the work, although that is often the case. Personal ambition, high economic aspirations, or inefficient use of time, are unacceptable excuses. Exoneration due to economic necessity should be extended only when supported by convincing explanations. Allowance should be made for short-term, unusual circumstances, e.g., a physician in training who has little or no control over his work schedule. The same person would not be excused if he persisted in excessive involvement in his work or career. Avoidance of interpersonal relationships or leisure activities for reasons other than devotion to work is not within the scope of the criterion.

2   Excessive devotion to work and productivity that usually prevents any significant pursuit of both leisure activities and interpersonal relationships.

1   Excessive devotion to work and productivity that occasionally prevents any significant pursuit of both leisure activities and interpersonal relationships.

Excessive devotion to work and productivity that usually prevents any significant pursuit of either leisure activities or interpersonal relationships but not both.

0   Denied or rarely or never leads to exclusion of leisure activities or interpersonal relationships.

adaptive traits, because they are irrelevant to a PD assessment. It also does not cover other (Axis I) mental disorders. There are instruments available for the evaluation of most of those conditions. We recommend their use prior to the IPDE, to provide the examiner with background information that is likely to enhance the reliability and validity of the questioning, probing, and scoring process. When it is not available from such an interview or from other sources, the IPDE examiner is expected to conduct a mental status examination and to take a psychiatric history.

The IPDE examines every subject for the presence or absence of all the PD criteria. It also provides a dimensional score for every subject on each disorder, regardless of whether or not they fulfill the criteria for the disorder. This additional information supplements that based on categorical diagnosis alone. Because PDs often reflect the exaggerated presence of traits that are continuously distributed in the population at large, the dimensional scores are not only useful to the clinician, but they also provide the research investigator with greater reliability and more versatility in data analysis.

Appropriate subjects

The IPDE is not intended for subjects below the age of 18, although with slight modifications some investigators have found it useful with those as young as age 15. The interview is not appropriate for those with severe depression, psychosis, below-normal intelligence, or substantial cognitive impairment. Whether it should be used with patients in remission from a chronic psychotic illness is somewhat problematic. For example, can one distinguish residual schizophrenia or the interepisodic manifestations of a bipolar disorder from a PD? A number of investigators have found the IPDE useful in studies of those disorders, and the decision is left to the discretion of the user.

Limitations of the IPDE

The IPDE is essentially a self-report instrument, and assumes that a person is capable of providing a valid description of disturbances in his personality. However, an individual may be unaware of some of his traits. He may also be resistant to acknowledging behaviour, if it is socially undesirable or if he thinks its disclosure is likely to adversely affect his best interests. This is especially likely to occur in patients who wish to terminate treatment prematurely, or in those about to be discharged from a mental health facility. Others may exaggerate disturbances in their behaviour. This is sometimes observed in those who are frantically seeking help, or who are dissatisfied with their treatment or the amount of attention they are receiving. It may also be a reflection of certain personality traits. Although subjects may also feign traits or behaviour, particularly in compensation cases and some forensic and military situations, the IPDE discourages this by requiring documentation with convincing examples, anecdotes, and descriptions.

Patients in a dysphoric state may have a selective recall or distorted perception of some personality traits. They may also confuse them with the symptoms of another mental disorder. There is evidence that the interest may be resistant to such trait-state artifacts in patients with mild to moderate symptoms, but additional research is required on this important subject. When possible, some investigators may wish to postpone the assessment until the symptoms of other mental disorders have remitted.

In ordinary clinical practice a family member or close friend is often used as an additional source of information to offset the limitations of the self-report method. We have experimented with various procedures for augmenting the subject's responses on the IPDE with data from other sources. Failure to acknowledge a behaviour, particularly one that is especially frowned upon by others, is sometimes followed on the IPDE by such inquiries as, 'Have people told you that you're like that?' Affirmative replies are then pursued with the question, 'Why do you think they've said that?' This approach can only be used selectively. If it were adopted in all situations where a behaviour has been denied, it would undermine the rapport between subject and examiner.

We have also tried a parallel form of the interview in which an informant was asked virtually the same questions about the patient. There were often discrepancies, and it was not always obvious who had provided the more valid information. It proved difficult to formulate a set of practice guidelines stipulating the source to be used in scoring a particular criterion. The problem is a complicated one, and a satisfactory resolution awaits the availability of more empirical data on the subject, including attempts to identify those criteria that tend to produce discrepancies, and characteristics of the subject and informant that might be used to determine the preferred source of information.

Meanwhile, the IPDE takes a practical approach to the informant problem with an additional scoring column for informant data. If the examiner has access to information from family, friends, mental health professionals, records, etc., that clearly contradicts the subject's responses regarding a particular criterion, then he/she may also score the criterion in the informant column provided two requirements are met. Firstly, he/she should have more confidence in that information than he/she does in the patient; and secondly, the other source must satisfy the identical scoring criteria that apply to the subject's response. Later, in entering ratings in the computer or transcribing them from the interview to the scoresheet, the scores based on the subject's report are bypassed in favour of those derived from the informant.

Examiner Qualifications and Training

The IPDE presupposes a thorough familiarity with the ICD-10 and DSM-III-R or DSM-IV classification systems of mental disorders, and considerable training and experience in making psychiatric diagnoses. Like other semistructured clinical interviews, its reliability and validity are inseparable from the qualifications and training of the person using it. It is designed for experienced psychiatrists, clinical psychologists, and those with comparable training, who are capable of making independent psychiatric diagnoses without a semistructured interview. It is not intended for use by clinicians in the early phase of their training, or by research assistants, nurses, and medical or graduate students. Most clinicians feel comfortable with the IPDE and achieve a basic proficiency after giving about 10 interviews. Those who wish to obtain the optimal training are encouraged to enroll in the course offered at the worldwide WHO training centres.

References

1. Jablensky, A., Sartorius, N., Hirschfeld, R. & Pardes, H. Diagnosis and classification of mental disorders and alcohol- and drug-related problems: a research agenda for the 1980s. *Psychological Medicine*, 1983; **13**: 907–21.
2. World Health Organization. *The ICD-10 Classification of Mental and Behavioural Disorders, Diagnostic Criteria for Research.* Geneva: World Health Organization, 1993.
3. American Psychiatric Association. *Diagnostic and Statistical Manual of Mental Disorders*, revised 3rd edn. Washington, DC: American Psychiatric Association, 1987.
4. American Psychiatric Association. *Diagnostic and Statistical Manual of Mental Disorders*, revised 4th edn. Washington, DC: American Psychiatric Association, 1994.
5. Loranger, A.W. *Personality Disorder Examination (PDE) Manual.* Yonkers: DV Communications, 1988.

Experiences with the IPDE

Alv A. Dahl and Antonio Andreoli

Personality disorders (PDs) have been considered among the least reliable diagnoses in psychiatry. When DSM-III PD diagnoses are made by clinicians, their reliability has proved to be rather poor.[1] The development of structured interviews for PD was, therefore, the natural next step in an effort to improve reliability. Loranger et al .[2,3] developed the Personality Disorder Examination (PDE) to fill that need. The IPDE evolved from the PDE, and includes the PDs in both ICD-10 and DSM-III-R. Its features are described elsewhere in this monograph.

After the completion of the International Pilot Study of Personality Disorders (IPSPD), the interviewers completed a questionnaire about their experiences with the IPDE.[4] At a meeting of investigators in Geneva in 1991, considerable time was devoted to issues raised by responses to the questionnaire. We will present the main findings and solutions chosen, since they reflect the dynamic process involved in the development of the final version of the IPDE.

Some centres sent a common reply to the questionnaire, while others provided the responses of the individual interviewers. They revealed a variety of experiences and attitudes towards the instrument and the problems in diagnosing PDs. They are reviewed question by question.

What is your general impression of the IPDE?

The overwhelming majority of the respondents found the IPDE to be a useful instrument for diagnosing PDs. One could perhaps argue that this was inflated, because they had a major investment in the instrument. But many of the sites had also tried other ways of diagnosing PDs in the ICD-9 and DSM-III classification systems, and they might simply have found the IPDE an effective way of doing it. Only minor modifications were suggested.

In the IPSPD the mean time of the interviews was two hours and twenty minutes. About half of the participants found that it took too long.

The investigators considered three solutions: (1) to administer the interview in two sessions; (2) to create separate modules for the ICD-10 and DSM-III-R PDs; and (3) to screen cases with a questionnaire with a low rate of false-negatives, thereby eliminating interviews with subjects unlikely to have a PD diagnosis.

Another question raised by some respondents concerned the duration of the behaviour used to define PD. ICD-10 and DSM-III-R do not specify the exact duration of the abnormal behavioural patterns constituting PDs, but both classifications use the term 'long-term'. ICD-10 states that the abnormal behaviour 'is stable and of long duration, having its onset in late childhood or adolescence,' while DSM-III-R says that it is 'characteristic of the persons's recent (past year) and long-term functioning (generally since adolescence or early adulthood).' There is some discrepancy then between ICD-10 and DSM-III-R regarding the onset of the maladaptive behaviour. The IPDE solved these problems by requiring that the behaviour associated with almost all the diagnostic criteria be present for at least five years, and at least one of the criteria be evident before age 25, in order to diagnose that disorder.

Concern was also expressed that a patient might have a disorder like depression that gives a distorted image of what he/she is usually like. A patient may also be unaware of some traits or unwilling to acknowledge them. The influence of depression is a well known problem in the evaluation of PD by self-report. A previous study with the PDE showed little influence of anxiety or depression on the categorical or dimensional assessment of PD.[5] It may be reasonable to conclude the same for IPDE if experienced clinicians carefully question the patients and use their clinical judgement. Severely depressed patients, however, might have difficulties in remembering their habitual state due to the effect of depression. An alternative solution is to postpone the PD examination until the patient is euthymic or to interview a relative. Lack of awareness or lying about unfavourable or less socially acceptable behaviour is a general problem in diagnosing mental disorders, and is not peculiar to structured interviews. Although the questions flow naturally, they presume that the subject is attentive, of normal intelligence, and motivated.

What are specific points with regard to applicability of IPDE in your culture?

Before the study several interviewers were concerned that the IPDE might reflect North American attitudes and social and cultural norms which may not be valid elsewhere. This criticism was not widespread, and ultimately the IPDE proved relevant across cultural and social settings.

Some investigators noted some problems of applicability. A few mentioned, e.g., that questions concerning reckless driving, and physical abuse of family members were problematic in their culture. Some high school education was probability necessary for an adequate understanding of the IPDE questions. And in some countries the high rate of long-term unemployment made the questions related to work experience less meaningful.

The following quotes illustrate experiences with the IPDE in different cultures:

The pattern of occurrence of personality disorders is largely unexplored in the Indian context, and the IPDE may usher in empirical investigation into this area.

Overall I am finding few problems of applicability of the IPDE to our culture of interest. Our subjects are mostly American urbanites who reside near the birthplace of the DSM-III-R itself. Therefore, one might expect that our subjects would share values and perspectives similar to those exemplified by the IPDE. This seems to be the case.

Respondents who were not psychologically-minded had great difficulty with borderline questions about identity. Although patients suffering from mental subnormality were excluded, those respondents whose intelligence appeared to be at the lower end of normal had considerable difficulty with these concepts. In contrast, subjects from middle-class backgrounds performed much more satisfactorily.

In French culture, people often answer not with specific examples, but more in terms of: 'I feel this way.'

It is my impression that the IPDE asks for a kind of psychological-mindedness or self-reflection which is often not found in Holland. I also think that the place of leisure activities and social relations compared to work is somewhat different in our culture, which could lead to an overdiagnosis of obsessive-compulsive personality disorder.

If there is need to shorten the interview, please indicate the sections that can be omitted.

All centres reported that the IPDE took a long time to administer, and the instrument can be shortened if only one of the two diagnostic systems is used. If only certain PDs need to be evaluated, it can also be shortened, but all PDs have to be examined to get complete differential diagnostic coverage. Several centres reported that they had not found any cases of DSM-III-R sadistic PD, and that the questions for that diagnosis could be omitted. It should be noted that in DSM-IV, sadistic, self-defeating, and passive aggressive PDs have been deleted, and this will shorten the IPDE significantly.

What do you think about the validity of the information obtained by IPDE (as compared to your clinical judgement)?

Most of the respondents reported that the validity of the IPDE was better than clinical judgement. Some patient denials and replies seemed doubtful to the examiners, and the IPDE does not allow clinical hunches. It may also be difficult to get valid answers to questions concerning items that are less socially desirable, e.g., the abuse of family members. The instrument assumes that the patient will be open and honest, but a number of patients with apparent personality abnormalities did not receive an IPDE diagnosis. It was not clear whether these patients were deliberately denying characteristics, or they had no insight into their own behaviour.

Do you think that the IPDE adequately covers information necessary to assess PDs?

The overwhelming majority of the respondents believed that the IPDE provided enough information to assess the PDs in DSM-III-R and ICD-10. A strength of the instrument is that it insures that all criteria are addressed. There is a question whether some of the questions are sufficient to elicit the necessary information. The impact of acute mental states may also be problematic, and needs to be assessed by examining the relationship with other mental disorders. To deal with this problem, the IPDE recommends the use of an Axis I instrument prior to the IPDE, to provide the examiner with the clinical information that is likely to enhance the reliability and validity of the questioning, probing, and scoring process. When it is not available from such an interview or from other sources, the IPDE examiner must obtain the information requested on the first page of the IPDE interview under the heading 'Background information'. Several respondents explicitly stated that information from an informant or from other sources was necessary for the diagnosis of PD.

What is your view of the IPDE interview on giving the interviewer a sense of satisfaction of completion?

Most respondents reported that they had comprehensively probed all the psychopathology of PDs. However, many also described a feeling of relief after having finished the interview, because they had been through a long and tedious task. Several reported a feeling of frustration, since they had collected a lot of information but did not know the diagnoses at the end of the interview. This required several additional minutes with a computer program, or even longer with the hand scoring algorithms.

Conclusion

A principal objective of the IPSPD was to field test and develop an internationally acceptable structured interview for the DSM-III-R and ICD-10 PDs. After the project, considerable feedback on the experience with the IPDE was provided. This chapter provides examples of that process, including some of the criticism. In the best tradition of international collaboration, these issues were discussed and acceptable solutions agreed upon by the participants in the study. The process persuaded us that the IPDE is an internationally acceptable structured interview for assessing the PDs in ICD-10, DSM-III-R, and now DSM-IV.

References

1   Mellsop, G., Varghese, F., Joshua, S. & Hicks, A. The reliability of axis II of DSM-III. *American Journal of Psychiatry*, 1982; **139**: 1360–1.

2   Loranger, A.W., Susman, V.L., Oldham, J.M. & Russakoff, L.K. The personality disorder examination: a preliminary report. *Journal of Personality Disorders*, 1987; **1**: 1–13.

3   Loranger A.W. *The Personality Disorder Examination (PDE) Manual*. Yonkers: DV Communications, 1989.

4   Loranger, A.W., Hirschfeld, R.M.A., Sartorius, N. & Regier, D.A. The WHO/ADAMHA international pilot study of personality disorders: background and purpose. *Journal of Personality Disorders*, 1991; **5**: 296–306.

5   Loranger, A.W., Lenzenweger, M.F., Gartner, A.F., Susman, V.L. *et al*. Trait-state artifacts and the diagnosis of personality disorders. *Archives of General Psychiatry*, 1991; **48**: 720–8.

Field Trial

Sampling, interviewers, interview procedures

Werner Mombour

Method of sample selection

The subjects of the study were in-patients and out-patients enrolled in 14 participating mental health facilities located in 11 countries in North America, Europe, Africa, and Asia (Table 1). The sites were selected to provide a broad representation of different nations, languages, and cultures. An additional consideration was the availability of experienced investigators with an interest in personality disorders.

Each centre was asked to attempt to enter approximately 50 patients in the study. To adequately explore the diagnostic utility of the interview an effort was made at each site to attempt to include approximately 30 patients with a personality disorder and 20 patients with a common mental disorder that was important in the differential diagnosis of personality disorders (PDs). The goal was to have an approximately equal representation of patients of both sexes between the ages of 21 and 55. Sampling of consecutive admissions was not feasible, and cases were selected at the convenience of the investigators. All patients were screened by experienced psychiatrists or clinical psychologists according to the following criteria.

Exclusion criteria

- Clinical evidence of toxic or organic brain disease.
- Moderate to profound mental retardation.
- Language or other communication difficulties preventing adequate assessment.
- Alcohol- or drug-use likely to prevent an adequate examination.
- Delusional disorders, acute transient, or other florid psychotic states.
- Evidence that personality functioning may have been significantly changed by another psychiatric disorder, e.g., psychosis.

Table 1. *Sites of International Personality Disorder Examination field trial*

Center	Country	Institution
Bangalore	India	National Institute of Mental Health and Neuro Sciences
Geneva	Switzerland	Institutions Universitaires de Psychiatrie-Genève
Leiden	Netherlands	Rijksuniversiteit te Leiden
London	United Kingdom	Institute of Psychiatry
Luxembourg	Luxembourg	Centre Hospitalier de Luxembourg
Munich	Germany	Max-Planck Institut für Psychiatrie
		Nervenklinik der Universität München
		Bezirkskrankenhaus Kaufbeuren
Nairobi	Kenya	Kenyatta National Hospital
New York	United States	Cornell Medical Center
Nottingham	United Kingdom	Stonebridge Research Centre
Oslo	Norway	Universitetet i Oslo, Psychiatrisk Institutt
Tokyo	Japan	Keio University School of Medicine
Vienna	Austria	Psychiatrische Universitatsklinik

Inclusion criteria

- The presence of a common mental disorder important in the differential diagnosis of PDs

  or

- Evidence of the following longstanding and persistent pattern of symptomatology and behavior which in the context of the given culture is considered an abnormality of personality due to the presence of:

(a) Markedly disharmonious attitudes and behavior usually involving several areas of functioning, e.g., affectivity, arousal, impulse control, ways of perceiving and thinking, and styles of relating to others.

(b) The abnormal behavior is enduring and not limited to episodes of mental illness.

(c) The abnormal behavior pattern is pervasive and clearly maladaptive to a broad range of personal and social situations.

(d) The above manifestations generally appear during childhood or adolescence and continue into adulthood.

(e) The disorder is of sufficient severity to lead to considerable personal distress and/or the disorder is usually, but not invariably, associated with significant impairment in occupational and social performance.

The screening clinicians utilized all available information on the patients and when necessary conducted their own interview. They summarized this information on a standard form that included a clinical diagnosis according to both their local practice and ICD-10.

IPDE training

Each centre (with the exception of Nairobi, where only one interviewer was available in addition to the screening personnel), trained at least two psychiatrists or clinical psychologists in the administration of the IPDE. The initial training consisted of a two-day workshop conducted at each centre by the developer of the instrument and co-ordinator of the project (AW Loranger). These training sessions made extensive use of videotaped demonstration interviews. Thereafter the principal investigator at each centre assumed responsibility for the training. Each interviewer was required to complete a minimum of 10 practice interviews before participating in the study. Scoring practices were also monitored during the study by circulating several videotaped interviews conducted in English.

IPDE interviews

To determine the interrater reliability of the IPDE, at each site an attempt was made to have 10 of the IPDE interviews observed and independently rated by another clinician. An effort was also made to have 25 of the patients at each centre reinterviewed with the IPDE by the same clinician several months later. The clinicians who conducted and observed the IPDE interviews were unaware of the diagnostic conclusions of the screening clinicians.

Clinical evaluation

The IPDE interviewer also conducted a general clinical evaluation of the patient. At several centers this included information derived from the following semistructured interviews: Diagnostic Interview Schedule (DIS)–Leiden (The Netherlands); Schedule for Affective Disorders and Schizophrenia (SADS-L)–London (UK); and Structured Interview for DSM-III-R (SCID)–New York (USA), Nottingham (UK), Oslo (Norway), Tokyo (Japan). After the completion of the IPDE, the interviewer summarized all of this information on a Clinical Evaluation Form.

Description of centres participating in the IPDE field trial

Aleksandar Janca and Charles Pull

Bangalore

Bangalore has been the capital of the southern Indian state of Karnataka (formerly Mysore) since 1830. The name comes from the word 'bendakalooru,' which means 'village of boiled grains' in the Kannada language. It is the fifth largest city in India, with about four million inhabitants consisting primarily of three cultural and linguistic groups: Kannada, Telugu, and Tamil. Bangalore was the headquarters of the British administration until 1881, and Britain retained its colonial and military presence there until independence in 1947. The city has an old section and several surrounding modern suburbs with many parks, wide streets, and a sprawl of military cantonments to the east. Often called the Garden City of India because of its salubrious climate, but more recently its rapid industrialization has also earned it the sobriquet, Silicon City.

The National Institute of Mental Health and Neuro Sciences (NIMHANS) is the largest mental health institution in the area and the largest postgraduate training centre in the country. It was established in 1974 as an autonomous institution, that amalgamated the Mental Hospital and the All India Institute of Mental Health. There are 24 departments grouped into three major sections: behavioural sciences, basic sciences and neurosciences. There is an 805-bed hospital with provision for 650 psychiatric and 155 neurological and neurosurgical patients. There is a multidisciplinary approach, which integrates service, training, and research in mental health and the neurosciences.

The Department of Psychiatry of NIMHANS has collaborated with the Division of Mental Health of the World Health Organization (WHO) for more than a decade. The collaboration has been particularly successful regarding the diagnosis and assessment of mental disorders and their culture-specific characteristics. Research investigators in the department have translated several diagnostic instruments developed by WHO into Kannada, Tamil, and Hindi, and participated in their field trials. The Institute serves as a WHO training and reference centre for the

Composite International Diagnostic Interview (CIDI), Schedule for Clinical Assessment in Neuropsychiatry (SCAN), and International Personality Disorder Examination (IPDE). In the IPDE field trial NIMHANS also served as a co-ordinating centre for several other institutions from which subjects were recruited. These were King George's Medical College, Lucknow; Institute of Psychiatry, Madurai; Madurai Medical College, Madurai; Jawaharial Institute of Postgraduate Medical Education and Research, Ponchiderry; K.E.M. Hospital, Bombay; Madras Medical College, Madras; and G. S. Medical College, Bombay.

Geneva

Geneva, the capital of the Canton of Geneva, is situated between the Alps and Jura mountains where the Rhône river emerges from Lake Geneva. Earlier in its history it was the centre of the Calvinist Reformation, and today it is a centre of commerce, trade, banking, and insurance. Geneva is the European headquarters of the United Nations and its related divisions, as well as the home of many other international organizations. It is an international city, two-thirds of whose inhabitants are recent immigrants about equally divided between those from other Swiss cantons and foreigners from all over the world.

Three public health institutions affiliated with the Department of Psychiatry of Geneva University Medical School provide mental health care to the adult population. Care is also provided by the emergency room of Geneva General Hospital and by approximately 160 private practitioners.

This study was conducted at the out-patient department of the Eaux-Vives Psychiatric Centre, which is responsible for a residential area with a population of about 115,000. There are specialized out-patient clinics for schizophrenia and mood and personality disorders, and a walk-in clinic for emergency psychiatric care. The out-patient department treats about 300 chronic and 500 new patients a year. Two-thirds of new admissions have severe anxiety, mood or stress-related disorders, and the remainder present with psychotic and depressive disorders.

The Eaux-Vives Psychiatric Centre is also a teaching institution affiliated with the Department of Psychiatry of Geneva University and the Clinique de Psychiatrie Generale I. The Centre has developed a research program focused on crisis intervention in acute patients, personality disorders (PDs) as predictors of outcome, and the cognitive functioning of patients with borderline PD and major depression.

Leiden/Delft

Leiden is situated at the confluence of the Old and New Rhine rivers in the western Netherlands. It was first mentioned in AD 922 as a holding of the Utrecht diocese. It developed around a twelfth-century castle and received its name (Lugdunum Batavorum) in the sixteenth century from Janus Dousa, a statesman and defender against the Spaniards. The University of Leiden was founded in 1575 and the city became a centre of Dutch Reformed theology, science and medicine. It is the birthplace of many famous Dutch painters including Rembrandt, Jan van Goyen, and Jan Steen.

The Department of Clinical and Health Psychology at the University of Leiden and the St. Joris Psychiatric Hospital in Delft participated in the study. Delft is a small city between Rotterdam and the Hague, famous for its handmade faience delftware. All subjects of the study were from St. Joris.

London

London is the largest port, and commercial and cultural centre of Great Britain and its Commonwealth. Founded by the Romans as Londinium, it experienced tremendous growth in trade and population at the end of the sixteenth century. Today it is one of the major centres of international trade and finance, and a tourist attraction for visitors from all over the world. Its museums, theatres and other cultural institutions make it one of the cultural capitals of the world.

The Bethlem Royal and the Maudsley Hospital, known informally as the Joint Hospital, have treated the mentally ill for more than 600 years. Today the Joint Hospital is administered as a postgraduate teaching hospital, and with the Institute of Psychiatry make up a tripartite organization commonly referred to as the Maudsley. The out-patient department serves some 3000 new attenders each year, representing all the psychiatric disorders. The hospital is responsible for a local catchment area in south-east London, south Southwark. In collaboration with the Institute of Psychiatry, the hospital has a wide range of specialty units, including those devoted to forensic psychiatry, alcoholism and the addictions, eating disorders, epilepsy, child and adolescent psychiatry, and neuropsychiatry. It is also a referral centre for specialist services for patients from all over the country. The Institute of Psychiatry is affiliated with the University of London and offers advanced training for psychiatrists, psychologists, neurologists, and other scientific and paramedical workers. It also conducts pioneering research to advance the understanding and treatment of mental illness.

Luxembourg

The City of Luxembourg (meaning 'little fortress') was built as a fortress on a plateau above the Alzette river, and was a natural defensive position for the Romans and later the Franks. Today scenic parks have replaced earlier fortifications on the western fringe of the old town. The city is an important financial centre and hosts several agencies of the European Community. There are highly diversified industries concentrated in the suburbs.

The Centre Hospitalier de Luxembourg is a general public hospital with a number of specialty departments. The Department of Psychiatry is one of the most active French-speaking WHO collaborating centres. It has been involved in many WHO research projects on the diagnosis, classification, and assessment of mental disorders. It has co-ordinated and tested the ICD-10 diagnostic criteria as well as numerous instruments developed by WHO. The hospital also serves as a training and reference centre for the Composite International Diagnostic Interview (CIDI), Schedules for Clinical Assessment in Neuropsychiatry (SCAN), and the International Personality Disorder Examination (IPDE). In addition to its use in the present study, the IPDE is used in the routine assessment of in-patients and out-patients with indications of a PD.

Munich

Munich is the capital of Bavaria and the third largest city in Germany. It traces its origin to an eighth century Benedictine monastery. Located on the Isar river it was founded in 1157 by Henry the Lion, Duke of Bavaria, who granted the monks the right to establish a marketplace (München means 'home of the monks'). Modern Munich is a city of great cultural and industrial importance, a major convention and financial centre, and one of the largest wholesale markets in Europe. Munich was represented in this study by the Max-Planck Institute for Psychiatry and the Department of Psychiatry of the University of Munich. A small number of patients from the Kaufbeuren mental hospital outside of Munich were also included.

The Max-Planck Institute for Psychiatry is a research institute for psychiatry and related basic sciences, and a 120-bed hospital. There are more than 1000 in-patient admissions a year, and an out-patient department serving about 2000 psychiatric and 2000 neurological patients annually. The in-patient department consists of an intensive care unit (locked ward), several open wards, a crisis intervention ward, and a neurological ward. Current research is focused on biological psychiatry, including neuroendocrinology and molecular genetics. There is also a great interest in the diagnosis and assessment of psychiatric disorders. The Institute has translated and tested a number of WHO diagnostic instruments.

The Department of Psychiatry of the University of Munich has an outstanding history dating back to Emil Kraepelin. It is now a part of the Munich Faculty of Clinical Medicine and comprises a 208 bed hospital, out-patient clinic, day and night clinics, and several affiliated department. Its staff comprises more than 300 professionals, including 97 physicians, psychologists, psychotherapists, and biochemists. The in-patient service cares for the inhabitants of Munich and its surrounding areas, and also admits patients from Upper and Lower Bavaria. It has 10 wards, including a research unit and one for the treatment of addiction. The out-patient department provides comprehensive care that includes a 24-hour emergency and liaison consultation service to the other hospitals of the Faculty of Clinical Medicine in Munich. There are also departments of neurochemistry, experimental and clinical psychology, psychotherapy and psychosomatics, neurophysiology and EEG, and forensic psychiatry. Patients are predominantly from working class backgrounds, but all socioeconomic groups are represented. They include mostly those with anxiety, depression, a history of suicide attempts, and personality disorders.

Nairobi

Nairobi is the capital of Kenya and one of the main trading centres in East Africa. The city was established at the end of the nineteenth century as a colonial railway settlement. It got its name from a waterhole known to the Masai people as Enkare Nairobi (cold water).

The city attracted many migrants from various parts of rural Kenya and became one of the largest cities in tropical Africa. It is the principal industrial centre in the country and the railway is the largest single industrial employer.

The study in Nairobi was conducted at three sites: Kenyatta National Hospital, Mathan Mental Hospital and the University of Nairobi Students' Health Centre. The Kenyatta National Hospital is the largest public hospital in the city of Nairobi and the majority of subjects for this study were recruited from there. The Mathan Mental Hospital is the largest in-patient facility in Nairobi with 1500 beds, most of which are occupied by patients with psychotic symptoms. It also has a 200-bed secure unit which houses mostly forensic cases. The University Students' Health centre provides medical services to students of the University of Nairobi and has about 40 admissions a week of cases with some psychological problems.

Patients of these institutions represent a whole range of sociodemographic strata, although the majority belong to the working class. Most of the patients from the forensic unit of the Mathan Mental Hospital manifest some PD characteristics, while the patients from the other sites most commonly show mixed anxiety and depressive symptomatology, often with a history of suicide attempts.

New York/White Plains

In 1609 Henry Hudson, an Englishman employed by the Dutch to search for a new route to the Indies, sailed his vessel Half Moon up the river that now bears his name. In 1626 the Dutch East India Company established a trading post on the present site of Manhattan, which they purchased from the natives for 60 guilders. It came under English rule in 1664 when Charles II seized it from the Dutch and gave it to the Duke of York. Situated on the Atlantic Ocean with one of the finest harbours in the world, in the nineteenth and early twentieth century New York was the gateway for most European immigrants to the US. Today, the city and its suburban communities has a population of more than 10 million, and is the financial, commercial and cultural capital of the US. With its unique ethnic mosaic it is arguably the most exciting and vibrant city in the world.

The New York Hospital and its affiliated Cornell University Medical College comprise The New York Hospital-Cornell Medical Center, a world-renowned medical resource for patient care, research, education and training. Chartered by King George III in 1771, it has accepted mentally ill patients since it opened in 1791 at the conclusion of the American Revolutionary War. The Department of Psychiatry maintains the Payne Whitney Clinic, a 100-bed facility adjacent to the main hospital in Manhattan, and the Westchester Division, a 300-bed hospital situated in a 200 acre park-like setting in suburban White Plains, where it has been located since 1894. Today White Plains has approximately 50,000 residents, and is a thriving shopping area and business community housing the offices and headquarters of many leading companies. It is also the governmental seat of Westchester County with its population of almost one million.

The Department of Psychiatry treats more than 10,000 patients a year in its in-patient and specialized ambulatory care programs. The patients represent the entire range of mental disorders, and reflect the ethnic and socioeconomic diversity of the region. The department has over 680 full- and part-time faculty members, who in addition to their clinical and educational responsibilities also conduct research on many of the biological and psychosocial topics on the frontier of modern psychiatry.

Nottingham

The city of Nottingham was established in the sixth century AD by the Anglo-Saxons who colonized the area by the River Trent and gave the settlement the name of Snotingaham (the 'ham' or village of Snot's people). Nottingham, the county town of Nottinghamshire, lies at the heart of the East Midlands coalfields and has extensive rail, road, and air connections with the rest of the United Kingdom and Europe. The population of the city and adjacent boroughs is approximately 650,000. Nottingham has two universities and is the centre for a wide range of artistic and cultural activities.

Nottingham's psychiatric services are divided into six catchment areas, each of which has a local mental health centre and an associated admission ward of 20 beds in one of two hospitals located in the north and south of the city. Patients in the study were selected from one of these sectors (East and Carlton), which has a resident population of 78,000 between the ages of 16 and 65. Those who required the services of the district-wide drug and alcohol unit or the rehabilitation and specialized psychotherapy units were not included.

All the psychiatric services of the East and Carlton sector are community based, with the exception of the admission ward. The psychiatric team is staffed by 1.5 consultant psychiatrists, three resident psychiatrists, one occupational therapist, five community psychiatric nurses, and four psychiatric social workers. The team operates from a purpose-built base which is located in the heart of the sector. It maintains very close links with the local community and is the first port-of-call for residents 16–65 years of age with mental disorders. There is no significant private practice in the area. Most psychiatric referrals are received from 53 primary care physicians in the sector. A smaller proportion are referred from social services, housing, and other agencies. The catchment area is located in part of the inner city and is subject to very high levels of social deprivation and unemployment compared to the rest of the city.

Oslo

Oslo, founded in about 1050 by King Harald Hardaake, lies at the head of Oslo Fjord in the southeastern part of the country. After it was destroyed by fire in 1624, Christian IV of Denmark and Norway built a new town farther west under the walls of the Akershus fortress, and called it Christiania. The population grew in the nineteenth century partly because of the absorption of surrounding municipalities, and it replaced Bergen as Norway's largest and most influential city. It was renamed Oslo in 1925 and today is Norway's capital, largest city, and home of its leading cultural institutions. Oslo also has the largest and busiest harbour in the country, and is the centre of Norwegian trade, banking, shipping and industry.

The study was conducted at the Psychiatrisk klinik, Vinderen, a clinic affiliated with the Department of Psychiatry of the University of Oslo. The clinic has primary responsibility for providing psychiatric services to approximately 80,000 inhabitants of sector-D west. This includes mostly the more affluent parts of the city, where psychiatric morbidity is less than elsewhere. The Psychiatrisk klinik works closely with general practitioners and the general hospital in the sector.

Tokyo

Tokyo lies on the Pacific coast of central Honshu Island. It has been inhabited since ancient times and was originally named Edo. It was renamed Tokyo ('eastern capital') in the nineteenth century. Today it is the capital of Japan and has a population of 12 million. It is the commercial, financial, and cultural centre of the nation. The locus of predominantly light and labour-intensive industries, Tokyo is also a transportation and international traffic centre.

The Keio University Hospital is located in Shinjuku-ku in the centre of Tokyo, surrounded by the beautiful garden of the Meiji Shrine and the Shinjuku Imperial Garden. It was established in 1917 under the leadership of Yukichi Pukuzawa, the founder of Keio University, and Shibasaburo Kitasato, the first dean of the School of Medicine. The hospital is affiliated with the Keio University School of Medicine, which was established in 1917 as part of the Keio Gijuku University founded in

1854. The hospital has gained a national reputation as one of the best medical centres in Japan. It has 1071 beds and serves over 3500 out-patients daily, more than 300 of whom are physician requests for consultations. Most patients are from the Tokyo area, but many come from elsewhere in the country.

The Department of Neuropsychiatry has 31 beds, 200 annual admissions, and a 30- to 40-day length of stay. Most patients have mood, neurotic, or eating disorders. The out-patient department has 10 new admissions daily and cares for 180–200 patients. The department has a reputation as a centre for both psychotherapy and pharmacotherapy. The majority of patients are middle class and come from urban or suburban areas, although some are referred from all over the country. As a teaching hospital it trains 10–15 new residents a year. It has trained almost 500 psychiatrists, about 10 per–cent of those in Japan. The facility also has a long history of research, particularly in psychopharmacology, psychoimmunology, psycho–oncology, and the quality of life of psychiatric patients.

Vienna

Vienna is the capital of Austria and home of 1.5 million people, nearly one-fifth of the country's population. It is located on the Danube river and is a gateway between western and eastern Europe. The mainstays of its economy are trade and industry. It is a city of vast cultural achievement, renowned for its baroque architecture and musical tradition. It was home to Haydn, Mozart, Beethoven, Schubert, Brahms, J. Strauss, Mahler, and Schönberg. Vienna was the seat of the Austro-Hungarian Empire until the beginning of the twentieth century, and the various states of the former empire have had a significant cultural and ethnic influence on this city.

This study was conducted in the Department of Psychiatry of the University of Vienna, part of a large university hospital located in the centre of the city. There are wards for general psychiatric and psychotherapeutic treatment. There is a small day hospital and an out-patient clinic that treats approximately 5000 patients annually. They are referred from all districts of Vienna and to a lesser extent from the eastern part of Austria. The national social insurance system insures free access to the hospital to the entire population. The subjects were recruited for the study from the out-patient clinic and psychotherapeutic wards. One patient was included from the day hospital.

Results

Armand W. Loranger

Course of the field trial

The first patients entered the study in April 1988 and the last subject was examined in December 1990. All record forms were returned to the project coordinator (AW Loranger), who verified them for completeness and contacted the centers regarding missing data or apparent errors in recording. The information was then entered in a computer at the ADAMHA data processing facility at Rockville, Maryland. In August 1991 the investigators met at the World Health Organization (WHO) headquarters in Geneva to review the results of the data analysis. At the meeting they also discussed the replies to a questionnaire that had been sent to all of the interviewers about the strengths and limitations of the IPDE, including its user friendliness, cultural relevance, and apparent clinical validity.

Patient sample

At the conclusion of the study, 716 patients had been examined, 243 reexamined, and 141 of the IPDE interviews rated by an observer. The average interval between the initial and repeat IPDE examinations was six months, with approximately 85% of the repetitions occurring between two months and one year. Table 1 provides the sample sizes of the subjects at each centre, together with the number of IPDE examiners. Table 2 contains information about the educational level of the patients. Their clinical ICD-10 diagnoses, exclusive of personality disorders (PDs), are presented in Table 3.

Personality disorder diagnoses

The IPDE personality disorder diagnoses in the DSM-III-R and ICD-10 systems are presented in Table 4. For the 243 subjects who were examined on two occasions, the diagnoses are based on the initial interview.

Table 1. Sample sizes and IPDE field trial centres

City	Centre	IPDE Examiners	Male	Female	Patients	
					In-patient	Out-patient
Bangalore	National Institute of Mental Health and Neuro Sciences	3	31	16	7	40
Geneva	Institutions Universitaires de Psychiatrie-Genève	3	11	21	2	30
Leiden	Rijksuniversiteit te Leiden	6	34	31	55	10
London	Institute of Psychiatry	3	23	29	26	26
Luxembourg	Centre Hospitalier de Luxembourg	5	28	24	46	6
Munich	Max-Planck-Institut für Psychiatrie Nervenklinik der Universität München Bezirkskrankenhaus Kaufbeuren	11	58	55	54	59
Nairobi	Kenyatta National Hospital	1	30	20	10	40
New York	Cornell Medical Center	10	48	52	56	44
Nottingham	Stonebridge Research Centre	4	26	24	0	50
Oslo	Universitetet i Oslo Psychiatrisk Institutt	4	20	28	20	28
Tokyo	Keio University School of Medicine	3	28	29	5	52
Vienna	Psychiatrische Universitatsklinik	5	27	23	14	36
Total		58	364	352	295	421

Table 2. *Educational level of patients at each centre*

Site	Percentage of centre sample years of education			
	<5	6–12	13–15	≥16
Bangalore	2.2	42.2	35.6	20.0
Geneva	0	58.1	19.4	16.1
Leiden	1.5	60.0	30.8	7.7
London	11.5	50.0	21.2	9.6
Luxembourg	2.0	58.0	32.0	8.0
Munich	0.9	64.6	22.1	12.4
Nairobi	32.0	61.3	6.5	0
New York	1.0	17.0	43.0	38.0
Nottingham	2.0	86.0	6.0	4.0
Oslo	0	64.6	20.8	14.6
Tokyo	0	32.1	23.2	44.7
Vienna	0	62.0	32.0	6.0

Tables A.1 to A.12 in the Appendix list the IPDE diagnoses at each individual centre. Table 5 presents the frequencies with which the specific DSM-III-R disorders occurred in the same patients. Table 6 provides the same information for the ICD-10 disorders.

IPDE interrater reliability and temporal stability

Intraclass correlation coefficients[1] were used to measure the examiner–observer agreement in scoring each of the 157 items on the IPDE, and their stability from the initial to repeat examinations. Since stability is influenced by the interrater agreement in scoring a single interview, correlations with a correction for attenuation[2] are included with the stability coefficients, to provide a more accurate estimate of stability *per se*. Table 7 summarizes these correlations. Tables A.13 and A.14 in the Appendix present the measures of interrater reliability and stability for each PD criterion in DSM-III-R and ICD-10, together with the frequency of occurrence of the criterion in the sample of 716 patients.

Table 3. *ICD-10 Disorders exclusive of personality disorders (N=696)*[*]

ICD-10 disorder (%)	No. of patients
Substance use (15.4)	107
Schizophrenia and delusional	
schizophrenia (2.3)	16
persistent delusional (0.6)	4
acute and transient psychotic (0.7)	5
schizoaffective (0.3)	2
Mood (affective)	
manic episode (0.1)	1
bipolar (3.7)	26
depressive episode (9.9)	69
recurrent depressive (8.9)	52
persistent mood (12.0)	77
other mood (0.2)	1
Neurotic, stress related, somatoform	
phobic anxiety (6.2)	43
other anxiety (13.6)	95
obsessive-compulsive (6.5)	45
reaction to severe stress and adjustment (5.9)	41
dissociative (1.0)	7
somatoform (2.6)	18
other (0.7)	5
Physiological disturbances	
eating (6.6)	46
nonorganic sleep (0.3)	2
sexual dysfunction (0.3)	2
personality disorder only (32.8)	228

[*]Includes multiple diagnoses in some patients. Diagnoses not available for 20 Nairobi patients.

Intraclass correlation coefficients were also used to measure the examiner–observer agreement regarding the dimensional scores, the number of criteria met on each disorder, and their stability from the initial to repeat examinations. These correlations are presented in Table 8.

Table 4. *IPDE DSM-III-R and ICD-10 diagnoses (N=716)**

DSM-III-R personality disorder	No. of patients	(%)
Paranoid	42	(5.9)
Schizoid	20	(2.8)
Schizotypal	25	(3.5)
Obsessive-compulsive	22	(3.1)
Histrionic	51	(7.1)
Dependent	32	(4.5)
Antisocial	46	(6.4)
Narcissistic	9	(1.3)
Avoidant	79	(11.0)
Borderline	104	(14.5)
Passive aggressive	36	(5.0)
Sadistic	2	(0.3)
Self defeating	9	(1.3)
+Not otherwise specified	92	(12.8)
Any personality disorder	366	(51.1)

ICD-10 personality disorder	No. of patients	(%)
Paranoid	17	(2.4)
Schizoid	13	(1.8)
Dissocial	23	(3.2)
Emotionally unstable		
impulsive	32	(4.5)
borderline	107	(14.9)
Histrionic	31	(4.3)
Anankastic	26	(3.6)
Anxious	109	(15.2)
Dependent	33	(4.6)
++Other	49	(6.8)
Any personality disorder	283	(39.5)

*Personality disorder diagnoses include patients with more than one type of personality disorder.

+Did not fulfill diagnostic criteria for any specific personality disorder, but met 10 or more of the 110 DSM-III-R personality disorder criteria.

++Did not fulfill diagnostic criteria for any specific personality disorder, but met 10 or more of the 56 ICD-10 personality disorder criteria.

Table 5. *Frequency of co-occurrence of DSM-III-R personality disorders in patients with a personality disorder (N=366)*

	PAR	SCD	SCT	ASP	BOR	HIS	NAR	AVO	DEP	OBC	PAS	SAD	SFD
PAR	**42**	4	5	8	16	13	1	9	3	4	8	0	1
SCD		**20**	6	0	2	0	0	5	1	0	1	0	0
SCT			**25**	0	6	1	0	4	2	1	1	0	2
ASP				**46**	16	10	2	5	2	0	9	1	0
BOR					**104**	26	7	18	16	4	16	1	5
HIS						**51**	7	8	10	3	9	0	2
NAR							**9**	1	2	0	3	0	0
AVO								**79**	14	7	12	0	5
DEP									**32**	3	4	0	2
OBC										**22**	5	0	2
PAS											**36**	0	4
SAD												**2**	0
SFD													**9**

Abbreviations: PAR, paranoid; SD, schizoid; SCT, schizotypal; ASP, antisocial; BOR, borderline; HIS, histrionic; NAR, narcissistic; AVO, avoidant; DEP, dependent; OBC, obsessive-compulsive; PAS, passive aggressive; SAD, sadistic; SFD, self-defeating.

Table 6. *Frequency of co-occurrence of ICD-10 personality disorders in patients with a personality disorder (N=283)*

	PAR	SCD	DIS	IMP	BOR	HIS	ANA	ANX	DEP
PAR	**17**	1	1	3	7	3	3	8	2
SCD		**13**	0	1	2	0	0	3	0
DIS			**23**	9	15	5	2	4	2
IMP				**32**	26	7	2	6	4
BOR					**107**	19	6	28	14
HIS						**31**	4	10	4
ANA							**26**	12	2
ANX								**109**	19
DEP									**33**

Abbreviations: PAR, paranoid; SCD, schizoid; DIS, dissocial; IMP, impulsive; BOR, borderline; HIS, histrionic; ANA, anankastic; ANX, anxious; DEP, dependent.

Table 7. *Interrater reliability and temporal stability of 157 IPDE items*

Intraclass R	Interrater reliability (N=141)			Temporal stability (N=243)		
	No. of Items	%	Cumul.%	No of Items	%	Cumul. %
0.90–1.00	13	8.3		0 (2)	0 (1.3)	
0.80–0.89	72	45.9	54.2	2 (13)	1.3 (8.3)	1.3 (9.6)
0.70–0.79	52	33.1	87.3	14 (42)	8.9 (26.8)	10.2 (36.3)
0.60–0.69	12	7.6	94.9	62 (62)	39.5 (39.5)	49.7 (75.8)
0.50–0.59	4	2.5	97.4	53 (27)	33.8 (17.2)	83.4 (93.0)
0.40–0.49	1	0.6	98.0	19 (5)	12.1 (3.2)	95.5 (96.2)
<0.40	3	1.3		7 (6)	4.5 (3.8)	

Kappa[3] was used to measure the interrater agreement and temporal stability of the PD diagnoses. Because of its instability in samples with an infrequent number of cases of a disorder, the recommendation was followed that it be calculated only when the prevalence of a disorder is at least 5%.[4] To provide more opportunities for the calculation of kappa, it was also determined by combining definite and probable diagnoses. The IPDE assigns a probable diagnosis when a subject meets one criterion less than the number required for the diagnosis. An overall weighted kappa was also determined for all PDs, including those with a base rate of less than 5%. It was calculated by weighing each category of PDs by the total number of cases assigned a diagnosis in that category by either rater, regardless of whether or not the raters agreed about the diagnosis. The numerator is the sum of the product of the diagnostic weight and kappa for each disorder; the denominator is the sum of the weights. The kappa values are presented in Table 9.

References

1   Ebel, R.L. Estimation of the reliability of ratings. *Psychometrika*, 1951; **16**: 407–23.

2   Nunnally, J.C. *Psychometric Theory*, pp. 219–20, 237–9. New York, NY: McGraw–Hill International Book Co, 1978.

3   Fleiss, J.L. *Statistical methods for Rates and Proportions*, 2nd edn., pp. 217–20. New York: John Wiley & Sons Inc, 1981.

4   Grove, W.M., Andreasen, N.C., McDonald-Scott, P., Keller, M.B. & Shapiro, R.W. Reliability studies of psychiatric diagnosis: theory and practice. *Archives of General Psychiatry*, 1981; **38**: 408–13.

Table 8. *Interrater reliability and temporal stability of IPDE number of criteria met and dimensional scores* *

Disorder	No. of criteria met		Dimensional score	
	Interrater reliability (N=141)	Temporal stability[†] (N=243)	Interrater reliability (N=141)	Temporal stability[†] (N=243)
DSM-III-R		*Intraclass R*		
Paranoid	.75	.58 (.67)	.85	.68 (.74)
Schizoid	.83	.72 (.79)	.86	.76 (.82)
Schizotypal	.82	.69 (.76)	.87	.81 (.87)
Obsessive-compulsive	.82	.75 (.83)	.89	.80 (.85)
Histrionic	.81	.75 (.83)	.87	.78 (.84)
Dependent	.89	.67 (.71)	.92	.72 (.75)
Antisocial	.88	.74 (.79)	.94	.92 (.95)
Narcissistic	.83	.71 (.78)	.90	.75 (.79)
Avoidant	.82	.71 (.78)	.89	.77 (.82)
Borderline	.89	.84 (.89)	.93	.87 (.91)
Passive aggressive	.92	.72 (.75)	.89	.78 (.83)
Sadistic	.80	.61 (.69)	.88	.76 (.81)
Self-defeating	.71	.74 (.88)	.79	.75 (.84)
ICD-10				
Paranoid	.78	.56 (.72)	.87	.66 (.71)
Schizoid	.79	.62 (.78)	.87	.74 (.80)
Dissocial	.88	.55 (.62)	.92	.69 (.72)
Emotionally unstable				
impulsive	.87	.74 (.85)	.89	.78 (.83)
borderline	.91	.82 (.90)	.93	.86 (.90)
Histrionic	.84	.69 (.82)	.88	.80 (.85)
Anankastic	.73	.74 (1.00)	.86	.77 (.83)
Anxious	.83	.74 (.89)	.88	.77 (.82)
Dependent	.88	.58 (.66)	.91	.65 (.71)

*Average interval between test and retest (temporal stability) was six months.
[†]For temporal stability, data in parentheses are corrected for attenuation.

Table 9. *Interrater agreement (κ), temporal stability (κ), and base rate (%) of IPDE DSM-III-R and ICD-10 diagnoses*[*]

Disorder	Interrater Agreement (N=141)		Temporal Stability N=243	
	Definite	Definite/Probable	Definite	Definite/Probable
DSM-III-R				
Paranoid	... (5%)	.51 (12%)	.24 (5%)	.28 (10%)
Schizoid	... (3%)	.87 (6%)	... (2%)	.68 (5%)
Schizotypal	... (1%)	... (3%)	... (3%)	.68 (5%)
Obsessive compulsive	... (2%)	.60 (6%)	... (2%)	... (4%)
Histrionic	.34 (6%)	.66 (13%)	.45 (5%)	.46 (12%)
dependent	.70 (5%)	.82 (9%)	... (4%)	.43 (9%)
Antisocial	... (5%)	.73 (9%)	.59 (5%)	.62 (9%)
Narcissistic	... (1%)	... (3%)	... (1%)	... (4%)
Avoidant	.71 (10%)	.78 (17%)	.48 (10%)	.56 (19%)
Borderline	.80 (10%)	.76 (16%)	.70 (13%)	.72 (19%)
Passive aggressive	... (2%)	... (4%)	... (3%)	.41 (6%)
Sadistic	... (1%)	... (1%)	... (0%)	... (2%)
Self-defeating	... (0%)	... (3%)	... (2%)	.71 (7%)
Any specific personality disorder	.59 (27%)	.70 (46%)	.62 (34%)	.63 (51%)
Overall Weighted Kappa	.57	.69	.50	.53
ICD-10				
Paranoid	... (2%)	.43 (7%)	... (2%)	.30 (8%)
Schizoid	... (1%)	... (5%)	... (1%)	... (3%)
Dissocial	... (4%)	1.00 (6%)	... (2%)	... (4%)
Emotionally unstable				
impulsive	... (4%)	.79 (7%)	... (4%)	.60 (7%)
borderline	.76 (12%)	.78 (16%)	.65 (14%)	.62 (15%)
Histrionic	... (3%)	.64 (7%)	... (2%)	.53 (7%)
Anankastic	... (2%)	.53 (6%)	... (2%)	.60 (7%)
Anxious	.72 (11%)	.77 (22%)	.64 (15%)	.65 (24%)
Dependent	... (4%)	.81 (13%)	... (3%)	.36 (11%)
Any specific personality disorder	.64 (25%)	.71 (43%)	.59 (29%)	.60 (44%)
Overall Weighted Kappa	.65	.72	.54	.53

[*]Kappa calculated only when base rate ≥5% according to both raters; base rates in Table are means of both raters. Average interval between test and retest (temporal stability) was six months. Probable diagnosis assigned when patient met one criterion less than required number.

Discussion and conclusions

Armand W. Loranger

This investigation represents the first attempt to assess personality disorders (PDs) worldwide with contemporary methods of diagnosis. The semistructured interview (International Personality Disorder Examination–IPDE), developed within the World Health Organization (WHO) program on diagnosis and classification, was designed to assess PDs within the framework and guidelines of two distinct but overlapping classification systems. DSM-III-R, which was intended for use in the US, is primarily the product of American psychiatric opinion, while ICD-10, which is meant for worldwide use, reflects the views and needs of the international psychiatric community.

Interrater Agreement

To provide a valid diagnosis an instrument must first demonstrate a reasonable degree of interrater reliability. An international test of reliability such as the present one involves patients from a wide variety of national and cultural settings, who speak many different languages. The examiners also consist of a large number of psychiatrists and clinical psychologists trained at many different facilities around the world. Therefore, this was an unusually exacting test of reliability to which no other interview for PDs has ever been subjected. The results, nevertheless, compare quite favourably with published reports on semistructured interviews that are used to diagnose the psychoses, mood, anxiety, and substance use disorders. Such comparisons, of course, must be viewed as rough approximations. There are obvious differences in the heterogeneity of the patient samples, the base rates of the individual disorders, as well as variations in the methods used to measure reliability. Furthermore, many of these studies have been conducted within one facility only, and rarely have they been undertaken outside the nation in which the interview was developed.

With these caveats in mind, we compared the results of the present study with those of the SCID Axis I field trial.[1] That study involved 390 patients at four locations in the US and one in Germany. The median kappa values for those individual disorders with a base rate of at least 5% were 0.64 for current diagnoses and 0.68 for lifetime diagnoses. In the present field trial, the median kappa values for the individual PDs (diagnosis definite) with base rates of at least five per cent were 0.70 in DSM-III-R and 0.72 in ICD-10. The overall weighted kappa values in the SCID study were 0.61 for current diagnoses and 0.68 for lifetime diagnoses. In the present study, the overall weighted kappa values for the definite diagnoses of the specific PDs were 0.57 in DSM-III-R and 0.65 in ICD-10. The median kappa values for an IPDE diagnosis that was definite or probable were 0.73 for DSM-III-R and 0.77 for ICD-10. The corresponding weighted kappa values for a diagnosis that was definite or probable were 0.65 for DSM-III-R and 0.72 for ICD-10. The SCID study did not identify probable cases.

The SCID study involved a test–retest design in which the interview was administered by different examiners at least one day but no more than two weeks apart. This is likely to result in lower reliabilities than when an examiner and observer rate the same interview, as in the present study. A similar test–retest design was not employed in the present study, because one of its objectives was to determine temporal stability over an extended period. There are practical and methodological constraints associated with the too frequent repetition of a lengthy interview.

The IPDE also fared well compared with other criteria-based interviews for PDs that have been developed in recent years.[2,3] However, reports of large-scale reliability studies conducted outside of the facilities where these other interviews were developed are rare or non–existent. The other interviews also differ from the IPDE in several ways. They do not provide coverage of ICD-10; they are not available in so many languages; and they do not have a detailed, item-by-item scoring manual.

Temporal stability

The term 'personality' refers to an individual's usual or characteristic rather than transient or situational behaviour. Therefore, a PD instrument should not only demonstrate interrater reliability, but it should also have temporal stability. Before imputing a particular criterion to a subject, the IPDE requires a minimal duration of five years, including some manifestation during the current year (past 12 months). Since the patients in the study were examined after an average interval of six months, temporal stability required that they provide essentially similar information on both occasions. The only exceptions were patients who might have failed to manifest the behaviour in both segments of the non-overlapping portions of the previous 12 months, or the rare patient who might have fallen a few months short of meeting the five-year requirement at the time of the initial interview. Naturally, these patients would adversely affect the measurement of stability. The determination of temporal stability is also influenced by the less-than-perfect reliability associated with the single administration of an instrument. Adjustments for that affect on the stability of the individual items, the number of criteria met, and the dimensional scores, were made by calculating additional correlations with a correction for attenuation.

There are comparatively few reports[4-8] on the temporal stability of the semistructured interviews that are used to make lifetime diagnoses of the psychoses, mood, anxiety, and substance use disorders. Table 1

Table 1 *Temporal stability of SADS-L diagnoses*[*]

Disorder	Andreasen et al.[4] (N=50)	Bromet et al.[5] (N=391)	Fendrich et al.[6] (N=69)	Rice et al.[7] (N=50)	Rice et al.[8] (N=1669)
Major depression	.75	.41	.54	.56	.61
Mania	.88			.48	.60
Hypomania	.06			.09	.33
Generalized anxiety	.15				.30
Phobic			.33		.34
Separation anxiety			.26		
Panic			.66		.37
Obsessive-compulsive			.66		.27
Alcoholism	.72			.73	.70
Drug use					.56
Substance abuse			.66		
Any diagnosis	.63		.62		

[*]SADS-L indicates Schedule for Affective Disorders and Schizophrenia-Lifetime version. All coefficients are k values except the study by Andreasen et al.,[4] which reported intraclass correlation. Four[5-8] of the five studies involved longer time intervals than did one[4] study. The time frame for those four studies were 18 months and 2, 5, and 6 years, respectively.

summarizes them for one popular instrument, the Schedule for Affective Disorders and Schizophrenia-Lifetime version (SADS-L). The findings indicate moderate, but at times disappointing, stabilities that are not consistently superior to many of those obtained in this study with the PDs. It should be noted, however, that four of the five studies involved longer time intervals than six months. The one study within that timeframe reported a kappa of 0.63 for the presence or absence of any SADS-L diagnosis. This compares with 0.62 in DSM-III-R and 0.59 in ICD-10 for the presence or absence of any specific PD on the IPDE. The studies in Table 1 did not report an overall weighted kappa, thus precluding comparisons based on that statistic. Another potentially relevant difference is that in most of these studies, the initial and repeat interviews were conducted by different interviewers. One study,[5] however, did not find significant differences in stability when the same and different interviewers were used; another study[6] reported an inconsistent effect.

There is very little literature on the temporal stability of criteria-based PDs diagnosed with semistructured interviews. There appear to be only three studies that involved more than a brief test–retest interval. One was based on an early trial version of the PDE,[9] which is no longer extant. The other two[10,11] reported on the stability of the Structured Interview for DSM-III Personality Disorders (SIDP). Pfohl et al.[10] repeated the SIDP in 36 depressed inpatients after 6 to 12 months. The kappa values, which ranged from 0.16 to 0.84, are problematic because of the small sample sizes of the individual disorders. Similar findings were obtained by van den Brink in the Netherlands.[11]

The belief that interviewers are perfectly interchangeable would seem naïve in view of the potential influence that the age, sex, and personality of an interviewer might have on the information provided by a subject. The assumption made by those who use semistructured interviews is that such factors ordinarily are not a major source of error. In planning the present study, consideration was given to a design in which half of the interviews would be repeated by the same examiner and half by a different examiner. This would have helped to determine how much the interviewers themselves, in addition to their rating decisions, contributed to the instability of the measures. However, concerns about scheduling and the availability of interviewers influenced the decision to use the same interviewers whenever possible. As a result, 93% of the interviews were given by the same examiner on both occasions.

A second interview, whether conducted by the same or a different person, may be contaminated by the experience of the first interview.

Repetitions can lead to boredom and decreased motivation. Patients may also believe that the interviews are no longer for their benefit but for that of the examiner. Repetitions can also produce fantasies that the interviewer is dissatisfied with the previous interview or is checking on the consistency of the responses. Patients may also refrain from providing as many positive replies as previously because of a heightened awareness that these invite further probing and prolong the interview. Elsewhere,[12] I have argued that the problem of attempting to measure the precise degree to which interviewers are interchangeable is reminiscent of the Heisenberg principle in physics: one cannot measure the phenomenon without somehow tampering with it in the process.

Another source of temporal instability is the possibility that patients in a dysphoric state may have a selective recall or distorted perception of certain personality traits. They may also confuse them with the symptoms of another (Axis I) mental disorder. An earlier version of the PDE proved resistant to changes in symptoms of anxiety and depression during the course of treatment.[9] In that study, the majority of patients had mood or anxiety disorders of mild to moderate severity. The finding has since been replicated with the DSM-III-R component of the IPDE (Loranger & Lenzenweger, 1992 unpublished). There is, however, a contradictory report based on a group of depressed patients treated with cognitive therapy.[13] That study used an earlier version of the PDE and the authors failed to specify the professional status and training of the interviewers, a potentially relevant variable. It may require an experienced psychiatrist or clinical psychologist to distinguish personality traits from transient pathological mental states and the symptoms of other disorders. The reliability and validity of the IPDE, like that of any semistructured interview, cannot be judged apart from the qualifications of the interviewers. At times, semistructured interviews have assumed a mystique of their own, and that caveat all too often ignored. The IPDE is intended for use by those who have the clinical sophistication and training required to make psychiatric diagnoses independently, i.e., without a semistructured interview. This is not to imply that the IPDE or any other PD interview is necessarily impervious to the influence of abnormal mental states, particularly those characterized by severe symptoms. We are encouraged, however, by the evidence that some clinical states do not appear to invalidate the assessment of personality. In any event, no attempt was made to determine the extent to which trait-state artifacts may have affected the stability of the IPDE in the present study.

Categories and dimensions

The prevailing systems of disease classification are categoric. They define the features of disorders, and ideally the categories have points of rarity with normality and other disorders. Although such nosologies sometimes fall short of the ideal, their value as shorthand forms of communication accounts for their widespread acceptance. However, proponents of what has come to be known as the 'dimensional' approach question the applicability of the categorical method to personality disorders.[14] One argument is that if PDs are not truly dichotomous in nature, reliability should improve with the use of dimensions because their measurement would incorporate more information than that provided by categories alone.

Critics sometimes overlook the fact that categories and dimensions need not be mutually exclusive, witness their harmonious coexistence in the classification of mental retardation and hypertension. Following that tradition, the IPDE was designed to provide categorical diagnoses and dimensional scores based on the categories. The results of the present study demonstrate the favorable effect of these scores on the reliability of the IPDE. This is illustrated, e.g., by paranoid personality, the disorder with the least stability. Although the DSM-III-R kappa was only .24, the stability of the paranoid dimensional score was 0.68 (0.74 with correction for attenuation). The stability of all of the DSM-III-R dimensional scores ranged from 0.68 to 0.92 (0.74 to 0.95 corrected), with a median of 0.77 (0.83 corrected). The corresponding correlations for the ICD-10 dimensions ranged from 0.65 to 0.86 (0.71 to 0.90 corrected), with a median of 0.77 (0.82 corrected).

These findings provide a striking example of the advantage of supplementing a categorical conclusion about the presence or absence of a specific PD with dimensional information about the traits that underlie the decision-making process. The IPDE dimensional scores include information about accentuated normal traits below the threshold required for a PD. A measure based on pathological traits alone consists of the number of criteria that a patient meets on a particular disorder. Table 8 (see chapter 'Results') reveals that this coarser measure is almost invariably associated with lower reliabilities than the dimensional scores, although the differences are not usually great.

Clinical acceptability and validity of the IPDE

At the conclusion of the study, a questionnaire concerning the IPDE was completed by all of the interviewers and discussed at length at the meeting of principal investigators in Geneva. The only significant reservation about the interview shared by a majority of the interviewers concerned its length. This was a necessary consequence of the decision to systematically inquire about all of the PD criteria in the ICD-10 and DSM-III-R classification systems. The mean length of the interview was 2 hours 20 minutes, and there was considerable variation around that figure. If a patient acknowledged many criteria, the subsequent inquiry for confirmatory examples and anecdotes prolonged the interview. If few of the behaviors were endorsed, then the IPDE went comparatively rapidly. If it became evident that the interview was likely to exceed more than one and a half to two hours, an effort was made to administer it in more than one sitting to prevent erosion of the quality of the interview from fatigue or boredom.

To offset the concern about the length of the interview and to make it more acceptable to a wider range of clinicians and investigators, it was decided to issue it in modules and to update the DSM-III-R component to conform to DSM-IV. While the longer version of the IPDE assesses all of the disorders in ICD-10 and DSM-IV, separate modules are available for those who wish to limit the examination to only one of the two classification systems. Those concerned with only certain selected disorders within one of the two systems can also restrict the interview to those items relevant to the disorders of interest to them.

A self-administered screening version of the IPDE is also available. It is not intended to substitute for the interview, because the literature indicates that PD inventories and interviews do not provide equivalent diagnoses. The screening inventory merely makes it possible to avoid interviewing those who are unlikely to receive a PD diagnosis on the interview. A field trial was undertaken with an early screening version of the DSM-III-R module in a sample of 258 university students.[15] The inventory produced few false-negative cases *vis-à-vis* the interview, but as expected it yielded a high rate of false-positives. Of course, the low literacy rate in some nations precludes its use with certain populations.

Whereas reliability refers to the consistency with which a diagnosis is made, validity refers to the accuracy of the diagnosis. The problems associated with establishing the validity of either an ordinary clinical interview or a semistructured one such as the IPDE are formidable. What should one use as the 'gold standard?' It would be meaningless to validate the IPDE against clinical diagnosis without first having established the reliability if not the validity of the clinicians themselves. If clinical diagnosis, as usually practiced, was 'as good as gold,' there would be no need to improve it with semistructured interviews.

A common practice is to invoke *construct* validity by demonstrating that a diagnosis agrees with that based on other interviews or inventories. However, this has restricted meaning, because the instruments usually sample identical content and often employ similar methods. The use of the so-called LEAD standard (Longitudinal, Expert, and All Data)[16] is also not without its problems. It is unlikely that many true 'experts' have the time or inclination to want to conduct a thorough examination and prolonged study of a large enough sample of patients to provide adequate representation of the various PDs and the differential diagnostic problems commonly encountered in ordinary clinical practice. The experts would also have to adhere to the same definition of a PD and diagnostic criteria, or there would be obvious artifactually based discrepancies. Inevitably the experts would also have to demonstrate how much they agree with one another.

The ultimate validation of the IPDE may prove to be a pragmatic one. Does the interview provide more replicable and useful answers to questions about etiology, course, and treatment than the assessments obtained from clinicians without benefit of the IPDE? The expectation is that it has the potential for doing so, because it is more likely to insure comprehensive, standardized coverage of the information required for a diagnosis. In theory the results of the examination should also be more generalizable and exportable than the clinical consensus of a panel of experts at one particular facility.

There are obvious cultural variations in what is considered maladaptive behaviour. Understandably one might question whether the PD criteria of DSM-III-R, which were developed for use in the US, are relevant or meaningful (valid) in other cultures. One might also wonder whether the ICD-10 criteria, which were designed for worldwide use, might be unduly influenced by Western psychiatric tradition. In the study no attempt was made to change the criteria themselves, in order to accommodate a particular culture. However, the clinicians were instructed to judge the meaning of the behaviour in the context of their culture. This did not prove to be a common occurrence. Examples include the DSM-III-R criteria pertaining to monogamous relationships (antisocial) and harsh treatment of spouses and children (sadistic). Surprisingly, the investigators at the various centres expressed few reservations about the applicability of either DSM-III-R or ICD-10 in their own nations.

Frequency of personality disorder types

The study had a very limited and specific objective, namely, to determine the reliability, stability, and clinical and cultural acceptability of a particular diagnostic instrument designed for worldwide use. In the absence of any prior evidence that PDs could be reliably and meaningfully assessed on a worldwide basis, it would have been premature and ill-advised to have broadened the scope of the project. The development of an acceptable instrument for case identification was a necessary prerequisite to any attempt at international collaborative or comparative studies of the PDs. The study was not intended to be an epidemiological survey of residents in the community or those under treatment. The sampling did not involve consecutive admissions, and there are obviously different thresholds associated with the request for mental health care in different cultures. Therefore, it would be imprudent to make too much of variations in the frequency with which the individual disorders were diagnosed at the various centres.

It is noteworthy, however, that most of the specific personality disorders in the two classification systems were observed in the 11 nations represented in the study. It is also of some interest that the two most frequently diagnosed types in the sample as a whole are disorders that were not included in either ICD-9 or DSM-II. They are borderline (DSM-III-R) or emotionally unstable, borderline type (ICD-10), and avoidant (DSM-III-R) or anxious (ICD-10). At least one case of these two disorders occurred at every centre with the exception of Bangalore, which did not report an avoidant diagnosis.

Two controversial disorders, sadistic and self-defeating, are not included in ICD-10, were relegated to the appendix of DSM-III-R, and do not appear at all in DSM-IV. Both were among the three least frequent diagnoses in the entire sample. Interestingly, the third, narcissistic, was not included in DSM-II and is still not recognized in ICD-10. It occurred in only 1.3% of patients in the study. This contrasts with passive-aggressive, which is not included in either ICD-10 or DSM-IV but was diagnosed in 5% of study patients and appeared in all centers except Bangalore.

Co-occurrence of mental disorders in the same patient

Not only did the majority of patients have other mental disorders in addition to PDs, but many also had more than one type of PD. Of the 366 patients with a DSM-III-R personality disorder diagnosis, 111 (30.3%)

had more than one personality disorder, including 55 (15.0%) with two, 32 (8.7%) with three, and 24 (6.6%) with more than three disorders. Of the 283 patients with an ICD-10 personality disorder diagnosis, 96 (33.9%) had more than one type of disorder, including 57 (20.1%) with two, 27 (9.5%) with three, and 12 (4.2%) with more than three disorders.

What are the implications of a patient having more than one form of mental disorder, particularly more than one type of PD? In some instances this may merely reflect the fact that two or more disorders share similar symptoms or diagnostic criteria. For example, substance abuse may be indicative of poor impulse control, a characteristic of antisocial, emotionally unstable or borderline PD. Similarly, social withdrawal is a diagnostic criterion shared by both schizoid and avoidant PDs. Another implication may be prognostic or therapeutic, with one disorder modifying the course or outcome of another. There is evidence, for example, that depression is less responsive to treatment, when accompanied by a PD. Comorbidity may also be a consequence of the fact that two disorders share similar etiologies. Finally, at times comorbidity may also be an indication of a defective or less than optimal classification system.

A fundamental problem in interpreting the meaning of the comorbidity findings from various studies, including this one, is that they are markedly influenced by the base rates of the disorders in the sample. These in turn are a function of the admission practices of the facilities from which the patients are drawn, not to mention the selection biases for inclusion in the studies themselves. Ideally, comorbidity should be determined from epidemiological studies based on probability samples from the community. Unfortunately these rarely if ever include a sufficient number of cases of most disorders, to provide definitive information about the true co-occurrence rates of the disorders in question.

ICD-10 and DSM-III-R

As previously noted, ICD-10 and DSM-III-R are different but overlapping classification systems. There are slight differences in nomenclature: anankastic/obsessive-compulsive, anxious/avoidant, and dissocial/antisocial. In ICD-10 borderline and impulsive are viewed as subtypes of emotionally unstable; schizotypal is located with schizophrenia and delusional disorders; and narcissistic, passive-aggressive, and the two disorders in the appendix of DSM-III-R, sadistic and self-defeating, do not appear. There are also several significant differences in the criteria in the two systems and some minor variations in their wording. Except for emotionally unstable, ICD-10 requires four of seven criteria for a diagnosis; and except for antisocial, DSM-III-R requires four or five from a list that varies from seven to nine criteria. Although there are fewer differences between ICD-10 and DSM-IV, many still remain.

A more detailed comparison of ICD-10, DSM-III-R, and DSM-IV is beyond the scope of this chapter. However, mention should be made of the extent to which ICD-10 and DSM-III-R tended to produce similar results in the present study. Within the limitations imposed by the sample sizes of the individual disorders, no statistically significant ($p<.05$) differences were observed in the base rates with which the corresponding specific PDs were diagnosed in the overall sample of 716 patients. There was a trend, albeit statistically not significant, for DSM-III-R to identify more cases of antisocial, paranoid, and histrionic behaviour and for ICD-10 to diagnose more cases of anxious/avoidant behaviour. Both systems provide a residual category for cases judged to have a PD that does not meet the requirements for any of the specific types. There is no method of identifying these patients without invoking some arbitrary standard. The IPDE assigns a residual diagnosis to anyone who does not meet the requirements for a specific disorder, but nevertheless accumulates 10 or more criteria from the various disorders. There are more opportunities to obtain the diagnosis in DSM-III-R than in ICD-10 because the former has 110 criteria and the latter only 56. It is not surprising, then, that approximately twice as many patients received a non-specific diagnosis of PD in DSM-III-R as in ICD-10 (12.8% vs 6.8%).

This, of course, does not address the question of whether the two classification systems actually identified the same patients as having a particular disorder. That can be determined by the kappa statistic, particularly for those disorders with a prevalence of at least 5%. There are only two of them; the kappas are 0.66 (borderline) and 0.52 (anxious/avoidant), evidence of moderate but far from perfect agreement. With the distribution of cases in the sample of 716 patients, these kappas were associated with 92% agreement regarding the diagnosis of borderline and 89% for anxious/avoidant. The kappa values for the remaining disorders should be viewed as relatively unstable because of the base rate problem. They range from 0.32 (dissocial) to 0.61 (anankastic/obsessive-compulsive), with a median of 0.52. The DSM-III-R and ICD-10 comparisons should not be affected by the less-than-perfect interrater reliability of the IPDE since the same examiner conducted the interview and rated the information on which the ICD-10 and DSM-III-R diagnoses for a particular patient were based.

The substantial disagreement regarding the dissocial and antisocial diagnoses is not entirely unexpected considering the different approaches the two classification systems have taken regarding the disorder. The DSM-III-R emphasized lawbreaking and criminal acts, while ICD-10 is more concerned with generic concepts such as lack of empathy, inability to profit from experience, and inability to maintain enduring relationships.

It is also possible to judge the overall agreement between DSM-III-R and ICD-10 for the eight disorders they share in common. This can be done by calculating an overall weighted kappa based on all of these disorders, regardless of whether they meet the criterion of a 5% base rate. That kappa is .54, an indication of only moderate agreement. There appears to be sufficient disagreement regarding the cases of personality disorders identified by ICD-10 and DSM-III-R to justify the prior decision of the WHO/ADAMHA (US Alcohol, Drug Abuse and Mental Health Administration) steering committee to develop an instrument that would accommodate both classification systems. The two, however, provide roughly similar interrater agreement and temporal stability when assessed by the IPDE.

Conclusions

The IPDE was administered by 58 psychiatrists and clinical psychologists to 716 patients in 11 countries in North America, Europe, Africa, and Asia. The interview demonstrated an interrater reliability and temporal stability roughly similar to instruments used to diagnose the psychoses, mood, anxiety, and substance use disorders. Experienced clinicians also found the instrument user friendly, culturally relevant, and clinically meaningful. By providing a standard method of diagnosis and case identification, the IPDE should stimulate international PD research, and facilitate comparisons of the results of such worldwide investigations.

References

1   Williams, J.B.W., Gibbon, M., First, M.B., Spitzer, R.L., Davies, M., Bonus, J., Howes, M.J., Kane, J., Pope, H.G., Jr. Rounsaville, B. & Wittchen, H.-U. The Structured Clinical interview for *DSM-III-R* (SCID), II: Multisite test–retest reliability. *Archives of General Psychiatry,* 1992; **49**: 630–6.

2   Stangl, D., Pfohl, B., Zimmerman, M., Bowers, W. & Corenthal, C. A structured

interview for *DSM-III* personality disorders: A preliminary report. *Archives of General Psychiatry*, 1985; **42**: 591–6.

3   Zanarini, M.C., Frankenburg, F.R., Chauncey, D.L. & Gunderson, J.G. The Diagnostic Interview for Personality Disorders: Interrater and test–retest reliability. *Comprehensive Psychiatry*, 1987; **28**: 467–80.

4   Andreasen, N.C., Grove, W.M., Shapiro, R.W., Keller, M.B., Hirschfeld, R.M.A. & McDonald-Scott, P. Reliability of lifetime diagnosis: A multicenter collaborative perspective. *Archives of General Psychiatry*, 1981; **38**: 400–5.

5   Bromet, E.J., Dunn, L.O., Connell, M.M., Dew, M.A. & Schulberg, H.C. Long-term reliability of diagnosing lifetime major depression in a community sample. *Archives of General Psychiatry*, 1986; **43**: 435–40.

6   Fendrich, M., Weissman, M.M., Warner, V. & Mufson, L. Two-year recall of lifetime diagnoses in offspring at high and low risk for major depression: The stability of offspring reports. *Archives of General Psychiatry*, 1990; **47**: 1121–7.

7   Rice, J.P., McDonald-Scott, P., Endicott, J., Coryell, W., Grove, W.M., Keller, M.B. & Altis, D. The stability of diagnosis with an application to bipolar II disorder. *Psychiatry Research*, 1986; **19**: 285–96.

8   Rice, J.P., Rochberg, N., Endicott, J., Lavori, P.W. & Miller, C. Stability of psychiatric diagnoses: An application to the affective disorders. *Archives of General Psychiatry*, 1992; **49**: 824–30.

9   Loranger, A.W., Lenzenweger, M.F., Gartner, A.F., Lehmann Susman, V., Herzig, J., Zammit, G.K., Gartner, J.D., Abrams, R.C. & Young, R.C. Trait-state artifacts and the diagnosis of personality disorders. *Archives of General Psychiatry*, 1991; **48**: 72–8.

10 Pfohl, B., Black, D.W, Noyes, R., Coryell, W.H. & Barrash, J. Axis I and Axis II comorbidity findings: implications for validity. In: Oldham, J.M., ed. *Personality Disorder: New Perspectives on Diagnostic Validity*, pp. 147–61. Washington, DC:American Psychiatric Press, 1991.

11 van den Brink, W. *Meting van* DSM-III *persoonlijkheidspathologie: Betrouwbaarheid en validiteit van de SIDP-R as II van de* DSM-III. Groningen: Drukkerij Van Denderen BV, 1989.

12 Loranger, A.W. Diagnosis of personality disorders: general considerations. In: Michels, R., ed. *Psychiatry*, vol 1 (chap. 15) pp. 1–14. Philadelphia, PA: JB Lippincott, 1991.

13 Stuart, S., Simmons, A.D., Thase, M.E. & Pillkonis P. Are personality disorders valid in acute major depression? *Journal of Affective Disorders*, 1992; **24**: 281–90.

14 Widiger, T.A. Categorical versus dimensional classification: Implications from and for research. *Journal of Personality Disorders*, 1992; **6**: 287–300.

15 Lenzenweger, M,F., Loranger, A.W., Kornfine, L. & Neff, C. Detecting personality disorders in a non-clinical population: Application of a two-stage procedure for case identification. *Archives of General Psychiatry*. (In press).

16 Spitzer, R.L. Psychiatric diagnosis: are clinicians still necessary? *Comprehensive Psychiatry*, 1983; **24**: 399–411.

Appendix

Table A1 *Personality disorder diagnoses–Bangalore, India (N=47)*

	No. (%) of patients	
IPDE Diagnosis	Definite	Definite/Probable
DSM-III-R		
Paranoid	1 (2.1)	1 (2.1)
Schizoid	2 (4.3)	2 (4.3)
Schizotypal	9 (19.1)	9 (19.1)
Obsessive–compulsive	0 (0.0)	0 (0.0)
Histrionic	1 (2.1)	1 (2.1)
Dependent	0 (0.0)	0 (0.0)
Antisocial	3 (6.4)	3 (6.4)
Narcissistic	0 (0.0)	0 (0.0)
Avoidant	0 (0.0)	0 (0.0)
Borderline	7 (14.9)	8 (17.0)
Passive-aggressive	0 (0.0)	0 (0.0)
Sadistic	0 (0.0)	0 (0.0)
Self-defeating	0 (0.0)	0 (0.0)
ICD-10		
Paranoid	0 (0.0)	0 (0.0)
Schizoid	1 (2.1)	1 (2.1)
Dissocial	0 (0.0)	0 (0.0)
Emotionally unstable		
impulsive	2 (4.3)	2 (4.3)
borderline	2 (4.3)	2 (4.3)
Histrionic	0 (0.0)	0 (0.0)
Anankastic	0 (0.0)	0 (0.0)
Anxious	0 (0.0)	1 (2.1)
Dependent	0 (0.0)	0 (0.0)

Table A2 *Personality disorder diagnoses–Geneva, Switzerland (N=32)*

IPDE Diagnosis	No. (%) of patients	
	Definite	Definite/Probable
DSM-III-R		
Paranoid	0 (0.0)	1 (3.1)
Schizoid	0 (0.0)	1 (3.1)
Schizotypal	0 (0.0)	1 (3.1)
Obsessive–compulsive	1 (3.1)	2 (6.2)
Histrionic	1 (3.1)	3 (9.3)
Dependent	0 (0.0)	1 (3.1)
Antisocial	0 (0.0)	1 (3.1)
Narcissistic	0 (0.0)	0 (0.0)
Avoidant	1 (3.1)	5 (15.6)
Borderline	4 (12.5)	8 (25.0)
Passive–aggressive	2 (6.2)	4 (12.5)
Sadistic	0 (0.0)	0 (0.0)
Self-defeating	0 (0.0)	3 (9.3)
ICD-10		
Paranoid	0 (0.0)	1 (3.1)
Schizoid	0 (0.0)	0 (0.0)
Dissocial	0 (0.0)	0 (0.0)
Emotionally unstable		
impulsive	0 (0.0)	0 (0.0)
borderline	5 (15.6)	6 (18.8)
Histrionic	0 (0.0)	1 (3.1)
Anankastic	0 (0.0)	2 (6.2)
Anxious	5 (15.6)	5 (15.6)
Dependent	1 (3.1)	6 (18.8)

Table A3 *Personality disorder diagnoses–Leiden, Netherlands (N=65)*

IPDE Diagnosis	No. (%) of patients	
	Definite	Definite/Probable
DSM-III-R		
Paranoid	6 (9.2)	11 (16.9)
Schizoid	1 (1.5)	5 (7.7)
Schizotypal	2 (3.1)	2 (3.1)
Obsessive–compulsive	3 (4.6)	5 (7.7)
Histrionic	3 (4.6)	7 (10.8)
Dependent	5 (7.7)	8 (12.3)
Antisocial	2 (3.1)	3 (4.6)
Narcissistic	0 (0.0)	4 (6.2)
Avoidant	7 (10.8)	2 (18.5)
Borderline	9 (13.8)	15 (23.1)
Passive–aggressive	1 (1.5)	3 (4.6)
Sadistic	0 (0.0)	2 (3.1)
Self-defeating	1 (1.5)	4 (6.2)
ICD-10		
Paranoid	1 (1.5)	4 (6.2)
Schizoid	1 (1.5)	4 (6.2)
Dissocial	2 (3.1)	2 (3.1)
Emotionally unstable		
impulsive	1 (1.5)	4 (6.2)
borderline	8 (12.3)	11 (16.9)
Histrionic	1 (1.5)	2 (3.1)
Anankastic	4 (6.2)	10 (15.4)
Anxious	9 (13.8)	18 (27.7)
Dependent	2 (3.1)	7 (10.8)

Table A4 *Personality disorder diagnoses–London, UK (N=52)*

IPDE Diagnosis	No. (%) of patients	
	Definite	Definite/Probable
DSM-III-R		
Paranoid	5 (9.6)	8 (15.4)
Schizoid	1 (1.9)	2 (3.9)
Schizotypal	3 (5.8)	5 (9.6)
Obsessive–compulsive	1 (1.9)	1 (1.9)
Histrionic	3 (5.8)	7 (13.5)
Dependent	0 (0.0)	3 (5.8)
Antisocial	9 (17.3)	10 (19.2)
Narcissistic	0 (0.0)	2 (3.9)
Avoidant	8 (15.4)	16 (30.8)
Borderline	10 (19.2)	13 (25.0)
Passive–aggressive	3 (5.8)	5 (9.6)
Sadistic	1 (1.9)	2 (3.9)
Self-defeating	0 (0.0)	2 (3.9)
ICD-10		
Paranoid	3 (5.8)	8 (15.4)
Schizoid	0 (0.0)	2 (3.9)
Dissocial	2 (3.9)	5 (9.6)
Emotionally unstable		
impulsive	5 (9.6)	8 (15.4)
borderline	12 (23.1)	13 (25.0)
Histrionic	1 (1.9)	5 (9.6)
Anankastic	1 (1.9)	3 (5.8)
Anxious	13 (25.0)	23 (44.2)
Dependent	1 (1.9)	4 (7.7)

Table A5 *Personality disorder diagnoses–Luxembourg (N=52)*

IPDE Diagnosis	No. (%) of patients	
	Definite	Definite/Probable
DSM-III-R		
Paranoid	3 (5.8)	8 (15.4)
Schizoid	2 (3.8)	5 (9.6)
Schizotypal	1 (1.9)	2 (3.8)
Obsessive–compulsive	2 (3.8)	5 (9.6)
Histrionic	4 (7.7)	9 (17.3)
Dependent	5 (9.6)	6 (11.5)
Antisocial	1 (1.9)	1 (1.9)
Narcissistic	0 (0.0)	2 (3.8)
Avoidant	8 (15.4)	3 (25.0)
Borderline	8 (15.4)	10 (19.2)
Passive–aggressive	2 (3.8)	2 (3.8)
Sadistic	0 (0.0)	0 (0.0)
Self-defeating	0 (0.0)	1 (1.9)
ICD-10		
Paranoid	3 (5.8)	4 (7.7)
Schizoid	2 (3.8)	3 (5.8)
Dissocial	1 (1.9)	1 (1.9)
Emotionally unstable		
impulsive	4 (7.7)	6 (11.5)
borderline	11 (21.2)	13 (25.0)
Histrionic	2 (3.8)	6 (11.5)
Anankastic	4 (7.7)	6 (11.5)
Anxious	13 (25.0)	17 (32.7)
Dependent	2 (3.8)	8 (15.4)

Table A6 *Personality disorder diagnoses–Munich, Germany (N=113)*

IPDE Diagnosis	No. (%) of patients	
	Definite	Definite/Probable
DSM-III-R		
Paranoid	12 (10.6)	25 (22.1)
Schizoid	4 (3.5)	9 (8.0)
Schizotypal	1 (0.9)	3 (2.6)
Obsessive–compulsive	5 (4.4)	15 (13.3)
Histrionic	15 (13.3)	20 (17.7)
Dependent	7 (6.2)	17 (15.0)
Antisocial	6 (5.3)	9 (8.0)
Narcissistic	4 (3.5)	9 (8.0)
Avoidant	14 (12.4)	25 (22.1)
Borderline	22 (19.5)	28 (24.8)
Passive–aggressive	6 (5.3)	9 (8.0)
Sadistic	0 (0.0)	3 (2.6)
Self-defeating	0 (0.0)	2 (1.8)
ICD-10		
Paranoid	5 (4.4)	12 (10.6)
Schizoid	2 (1.8)	5 (4.5)
Dissocial	2 (1.8)	6 (5.3)
Emotionally unstable		
impulsive	8 (7.1)	15 (13.3)
borderline	20 (17.7)	26 (23.0)
Histrionic	11 (9.7)	18 (15.9)
Anankastic	6 (5.3)	14 (12.4)
Anxious	15 (13.3)	28 (24.8)
Dependent	10 (8.8)	23 (20.4)

Table A7 *Personality disorder diagnoses–Nairobi, Kenya (N=50)*

IPDE Diagnosis	No. (%) of patients	
	Definite	Definite/Probable
DSM-III-R		
Paranoid	2 (4.0)	3 (6.0)
Schizoid	6 (12.0)	11 (22.0)
Schizotypal	4 (8.0)	7 (14.0)
Obsessive–compulsive	3 (6.0)	4 (8.0)
Histrionic	4 (8.0)	5 (10.0)
Dependent	3 (6.0)	5 (10.0)
Antisocial	8 (16.0)	11 (22.0)
Narcissistic	0 (0.0)	2 (4.0)
Avoidant	7 (14.0)	12 (24.0)
Borderline	0 (0.0)	5 (10.0)
Passive–aggressive	12 (24.0)	16 (32.0)
Sadistic	1 (2.0)	1 (2.0)
Self-defeating	0 (0.0)	0 (0.0)
ICD-10		
Paranoid	2 (4.0)	4 (8.0)
Schizoid	5 (10.0)	8 (16.0)
Dissocial	5 (10.0)	7 (14.0)
Emotionally unstable		
impulsive	2 (4.0)	4 (8.0)
borderline	4 (8.0)	5 (10.0)
Histrionic	5 (10.0)	7 (14.0)
Anankastic	3 (6.0)	4 (8.0)
Anxious	8 (16.0)	11 (22.0)
Dependent	3 (6.0)	5 (10.0)

Table 8A *Personality disorder diagnoses–New York, USA (N=100)*

IPDE Diagnosis	No. (%) of patients	
	Definite	Definite/Probable
DSM-III-R		
Paranoid	2 (2.0)	6 (6.0)
Schizoid	1 (1.0)	3 (3.0)
Schizotypal	1 (1.0)	2 (2.0)
Obsessive–compulsive	0 (0.0)	1 (1.0)
Histrionic	8 (8.0)	17 (17.0)
Dependent	2 (2.0)	7 (7.0)
Antisocial	2 (2.0)	5 (5.0)
Narcissistic	2 (2.0)	8 (8.0)
Avoidant	7 (7.0)	13 (13.0)
Borderline	15 (15.0)	20 (20.0)
Passive–aggressive	5 (5.0)	10 (10.0)
Sadistic	0 (0.0)	2 (2.0)
Self-defeating	1 (1.0)	6 (6.0)
ICD-10		
Paranoid	0 (0.0)	4 (4.0)
Schizoid	0 (0.0)	2 (2.0)
Dissocial	4 (4.0)	6 (6.0)
Emotionally unstable		
impulsive	1 (1.0)	4 (4.0)
borderline	16 (16.0)	19 (19.0)
Histrionic	3 (3.0)	9 (9.0)
Anankastic	1 (1.0)	4 (4.0)
Anxious	10 (10.0)	14 (14.0)
Dependent	1 (1.0)	7 (7.0)

Table A9 *Personality disorder diagnoses–Nottingham, UK (N=50)*

	No. (%) of patients	
IPDE Diagnosis	Definite	Definite/Probable
DSM-III-R		
Paranoid	5 (10.0)	8 (16.0)
Schizoid	3 (6.0)	4 (8.0)
Schizotypal	1 (2.0)	2 (4.0)
Obsessive–compulsive	1 (2.0)	1 (2.0)
Histrionic	2 (4.0)	3 (6.0)
Dependent	1 (2.0)	3 (6.0)
Antisocial	3 (6.0)	9 (18.0)
Narcissistic	0 (0.0)	0 (0.0)
Avoidant	4 (8.0)	8 (16.0)
Borderline	5 (10.0)	6 (12.0)
Passive–aggressive	1 (2.0)	2 (4.0)
Sadistic	0 (0.0)	0 (0.0)
Self-defeating	1 (2.0)	1 (2.0)
ICD-10		
Paranoid	1 (2.0)	10 (20.0)
Schizoid	1 (2.0)	3 (6.0)
Dissocial	2 (4.0)	5 (10.0)
Emotionally unstable		
impulsive	1 (2.0)	4 (8.0)
borderline	6 (12.0)	6 (12.0)
Histrionic	0 (0.0)	0 (0.0)
Anankastic	1 (2.0)	3 (6.0)
Anxious	7 (14.0)	15 (30.0)
Dependent	1 (2.0)	3 (6.0)

Table A10 *Personality disorder diagnoses–Oslo, Norway (N=48)*

IPDE Diagnosis	No. (%) of patients	
	Definite	Definite/Probable
DSM-III-R		
Paranoid	2 (4.2)	6 (12.5)
Schizoid	0 (0.0)	0 (0.0)
Schizotypal	1 (2.1)	1 (2.1)
Obsessive–compulsive	1 (2.1)	2 (4.2)
Histrionic	4 (8.3)	7 (14.6)
Dependent	4 (8.3)	8 (16.7)
Antisocial	5 (10.4)	9 (18.8)
Narcissistic	1 (2.1)	1 (2.1)
Avoidant	5 (10.4)	9 (18.8)
Borderline	10 (20.8)	16 (39.6)
Passive–aggressive	1 (2.1)	1 (2.1)
Sadistic	0 (0.0)	2 (4.2)
Self-defeating	2 (4.2)	2 (4.2)
ICD-10		
Paranoid	0 (0.0)	8 (16.7)
Schizoid	0 (0.0)	0 (0.0)
Dissocial	1 (2.1)	1 (2.1)
Emotionally unstable		
impulsive	4 (8.3)	5 (10.4)
borderline	11 (22.9)	13 (27.1)
Histrionic	4 (8.3)	6 (12.5)
Anankastic	3 (6.3)	7 (14.6)
Anxious	7 (14.6)	13 (27.1)
Dependent	5 (10.4)	8 (16.7)

Table A11 *Personality disorder diagnoses–Tokyo, Japan (N=57)*

IPDE Diagnosis	No. (%) of patients	
	Definite	Definite/Probable
DSM-III-R		
Paranoid	2 (3.5)	4 (7.0)
Schizoid	0 (0.0)	3 (5.3)
Schizotypal	1 (1.8)	3 (5.3)
Obsessive–compulsive	2 (3.5)	7 (12.3)
Histrionic	2 (3.5)	6 (10.5)
Dependent	1 (1.8)	3 (5.3)
Antisocial	0 (0.0)	1 (1.8)
Narcissistic	1 (1.8)	2 (3.5)
Avoidant	6 (10.5)	10 (17.5)
Borderline	4 (7.0)	4 (7.0)
Passive–aggressive	1 (1.8)	3 (5.3)
Sadistic	0 (0.0)	0 (0.0)
Self-defeating	0 (0.0)	0 (0.0)
ICD-10		
Paranoid	1 (1.8)	6 (10.5)
Schizoid	1 (1.8)	1 (1.8)
Dissocial	0 (0.0)	0 (0.0)
Emotionally unstable		
impulsive	0 (0.0)	1 (1.8)
borderline	4 (7.0)	5 (8.8)
Histrionic	2 (3.5)	3 (5.3)
Anankastic	2 (3.5)	5 (8.8)
Anxious	10 (17.5)	21 (36.8)
Dependent	0 (0.0)	4 (7.0)

Table A12 *Personality disorder diagnoses–Vienna, Austria (N=50)*

	No. (%) of patients	
IPDE Diagnosis	Definite	Definite/Probable
DSM-III-R		
Paranoid	2 (4.0)	2 (4.0)
Schizoid	1 (2.0)	3 (6.0)
Schizotypal	2 (4.0)	3 (6.0)
Obsessive–compulsive	3 (6.0)	6 (12.0)
Histrionic	4 (8.0)	10 (20.0)
Dependent	4 (8.0)	12 (24.0)
Antisocial	2 (4.0)	5 (10.0)
Narcissistic	1 (2.0)	1 (2.0)
Avoidant	12 (24.0)	18 (36.0)
Borderline	10 (20.0)	14 (28.0)
Passive–aggressive	2 (4.0)	4 (8.0)
Sadistic	0 (0.0)	1 (2.0)
Self-defeating	4 (8.0)	7 (14.0)
ICD-10		
Paranoid	1 (2.0)	4 (8.0)
Schizoid	0 (0.0)	2 (4.0)
Dissocial	4 (8.0)	8 (16.0)
Emotionally unstable		
impulsive	4 (8.0)	5 (10.0)
borderline	10 (20.0)	10 (20.0)
Histrionic	2 (4.0)	6 (12.0)
Anankastic	1 (2.0)	9 (18.0)
Anxious	12 (24.0)	19 (38.0)
Dependent	7 (14.0)	11 (22.0)

Table A13 *Frequency of occurrence, interrater reliability and stability of DSM-III-R criteria*

Criterion	Frequency of occurrence (%) N=726	Reliability (R) N=151	Stability (R) N=243*	
Paranoid				
1	10	.70	.56	(.67)
2	16	.79	.59	(.66)
3	12	.81	.54	(.60)
4	21	.79	.56	(.63)
5	13	.75	.31	(.36)
6	17	.77	.49	(.56)
7	8	.77	.62	(.71)
Schizoid				
1	6	.71	.39	(.46)
2	21	.83	.68	(.75)
3	5	.74	.38	(.44)
4	9	.76	.49	(.56)
5	2	.33	.36	(.63)
6	22	.77	.63	(.72)
7	4	.57	.60	(.80)
Schizotypal				
1	18	.83	.63	(.69)
2	23	.86	.70	(.75)
3	10	.78	.66	(.75)
4	9	.86	.60	(.64)
5	2	.32	.63	(1.1)
6	22	.77	.63	(.72)
7	2	.79	.65	(.73)
8	3	.68	.64	(.78)
9	4	.72	.60	(.71)
Antisocial				
B1	14	.86	.85	(.91)
B2	9	.87	.74	(.80)
B3	8	.82	.77	(.85)
B4	3	1.00	.51	(.51)
B5	1	00	.47	(0)
B6	3	.74	.59	(.69)

Table A13 (*cont*)

Criterion	Frequency of occurrence (%) N=726	Reliability (R) N=151	Stability (R) N=243*	
B7	3	.89	.49	(.52)
B8	4	.93	.60	(.62)
B9	2	.73	.65	(.76)
B10	11	.89	.65	(.69)
B11	12	.84	.72	(.78)
B12	1	.89	00	(0)
C1	12	.82	.64	(.93)
C2	17	.86	.80	(.86)
C3	15	.86	.68	(.73)
C4	10	.81	.75	(.83)
C5	7	.74	.71	(.83)
C6	11	.78	.67	(.76)
C7	19	.87	.71	(.76)
C8	6	.86	.63	(.68)
C9	8	.55	.47	(.64)
C10	9	.73	.59	(.69)
Borderline				
1	17	.89	.65	(.69)
2	26	.86	.77	(.83)
3	28	.84	.59	(.64)
4	22	.81	.64	(.71)
5	27	.79	.79	(.89)
6	15	.74	.64	(.74)
7	28	.83	.68	(.75)
8	12	.82	.43	(.47)
Histrionic				
1	15	.82	.56	(.62)
2	5	.62	.47	(.59)
3	10	.79	.54	(.61)
4	10	.91	.75	(.79)
5	12	.88	.60	(.64)
6	18	.79	.60	(.67)
7	20	.77	.62	(.70)
8	3	.70	.56	(.67)

Table A13 (*cont*)

Criterion	Frequency of occurrence (%) N=726	Reliability (R) N=151	Stability (R) N=243*	
Narcissistic				
1	23	.74	.61	(.71)
2	10	.85	.54	(.59)
3	7	.61	.51	(.65)
4	12	.77	.56	(.64)
5	12	.74	.56	(.65)
6	6	.74	.55	(.64)
7	12	.83	.56	(.61)
8	7	.89	.58	(.62)
9	8	.89	.52	(.55)
Avoidant				
1	33	.82	.63	(.69)
2	22	.77	.63	(.72)
3	20	.80	.48	(.54)
4	17	.89	.56	(.59)
5	18	.69	.58	(.70)
6	21	.91	.70	(.74)
7	13	.71	.50	(.60)
Dependent				
1	11	.86	.52	(.56)
2	10	.87	.57	(.61)
3	7	.84	.41	(.45)
4	10	.89	.65	(.69)
5	8	.62	.69	(.87)
6	14	.90	.45	(.47)
7	24	.87	.47	(.50)
8	18	.91	.50	(.53)
9	33	.82	.63	(.69)
Obsessive–compulsive				
1	15	.90	.48	(.50)
2	10	.84	.57	(.62)
3	14	.78	.58	(.66)
4	13	.90	.53	(.56)
5	23	.78	.62	(.70)

Table A13 (*cont*)

Criterion	Frequency of occurrence (%) N=726	Reliability (R) N=151	Stability (R) N=243*	
6	10	.76	.55	(.63)
7	19	.82	0	(0)
8	4	.72	.54	(.64)
9	10	.85	.71	(.77)
Passive–aggressive				
1	15	.80	.56	(.63)
2	19	.91	.63	(.66)
3	10	.84	.63	(.68)
4	6	.85	.47	(.51)
5	8	.77	.54	(.61)
6	8	.86	.58	(.62)
7	12	.68	.55	(.65)
8	6	.76	.58	(.67)
9	12	.77	.68	(.77)
Sadistic				
1	2	.67	.26	(.32)
2	2	.86	.56	(.60)
3	2	.51	.40	(.56)
4	2	.72	.52	(.61)
5	3	.90	.50	(.53)
6	6	.65	.65	(.81)
7	4	.76	.40	(.46)
8	3	.77	.69	(.79)
Self-defeating				
1	14	.88	.67	(.71)
2	15	.80	.51	(.57)
3	6	.83	.62	(.68)
4	8	.73	.59	(.69)
5	7	.48	.46	(.67)
6	12	.80	.56	(.63)
7	7	.81	.61	(.68)
8	12	.61	.56	(.72)

*For temporal stability data in parentheses are corrected for attentuation

Table A14 *Frequency of occurrence, interrater reliability and stability of ICD-10 criteria*

Criterion	IPDE Item	Frequency of Occurrence (%) N=726	Reliability (R) N=151	Stability (R) N=243*	
Paranoid					
1	90	20	.79	.48	(.54)
2	82	21	.79	.56	(.63)
3	85,157	7	.71	.58	(.69)
4	67	11	.79	.56	(.63)
5	119	8	.77	.62	(.71)
6	86	18	.83	.63	(.69)
7	121	5	.75	.55	(.64)
Schizoid					
1	96	6	.69	.45	(.54)
2	93,101,155	10	.72	.30	(.35)
3	87	2	.33	.36	(.63)
4	114	9	.76	.49	(.56)
5	45,51	18	.78	.66	(.75)
6	48	22	.77	.63	(.72)
7	154	2	.32	.63	(1.1)
Dissocial					
1	63	7	.89	.58	(.62)
2	136	15	.84	.73	(.80)
3	50	12	.66	.60	(.74)
4	34,129	17	.80	.65	(.73)
5	137,139	9	.78	.60	(.68)
6	138	10	.81	.58	(.64)
7	98	15	.86	.64	(.69)
Impulsive					
1	125	17	.82	.64	(.71)
2	124	16	.85	.68	(.74)
3	106	28	.84	.59	(.64
4	99,116	13	.67	.64	(.78)
5	100	15	.81	.57	.63)
6	66	11	.79	.68	(.76)
7	27	17	.80	.62	(.69)

Table A14 (*cont.*)

Criterion	IPDE Item	Frequency of Occurrence (%) N=726	Reliability (R) N=151	Stability (R) N=243[*]	
Histrionic					
1	94	10	.91	.75	(.79)
2	28	14	.90	.53	(.56)
3	105	18	.79	.60	(.68)
4	35	16	.76	.62	(.71)
5	38,88	23	.80	.57	(.64)
6	1,33	12	.83	.54	(.59)
7	62	10	.85	.54	(.59)
Anankastic					
1	23	23	.78	.62	(.70)
2	2,3,4	12	.86	.52	(.56)
3	1,33	12	.83	.54	(.59)
4	93	19	.82	0	(0)
5	60	14	.78	.58	(.66)
6	108	16	.75	.47	(.54)
7	31	9	.78	.63	(.71)
Anxious					
1	107	32	.88	.62	(.66)
2	30	28	.85	.67	(.73)
3	40	20	.90	.60	(.63)
4	56,88	29	.86	.62	(.69)
5	55	20	.80	.48	(.54)
6	111	13	.71	.50	(.59)
7	110	22	.83	.57	(.63)
Dependent					
1	24	10	.87	.57	(.61)
2	76	26	.81	.60	(.67)
3	75	18	.88	.49	(.52)
4	29	14	.81	.65	(.72)
5	104,112	16	.90	.48	(.50)
6	57	24	.87	.47	(.50)
7	25	14	.84	.64	(.70)

[*] For temporal stability data in parentheses are corrected for attentuation

II   International Personality Disorder Examination (IPDE)

ICD-10 Module

112

Acknowledgements

The IPDE was developed for the World Health Organization (WHO) by Dr. Armand W. Loranger in collaboration with the following colleagues from the international psychiatric community: Drs. Antonio Andreoli (Geneva), Peter Berger (Vienna), Peter Buchheim (Munich), S. M. Channabasavanna (Bangalore), Bina Coid (London), Alv A. Dahl (Oslo), Rene F. W. Diekstra (Leiden), Brian Ferguson (Nottingham), Lawrence B. Jacobsberg (New York), Aleksandar Janca (WHO), Werner Mombour (Munich), Yutaka Ono (Tokyo), Charles Pull (Luxembourg), Norman Sartorius (Geneva), and R. Onyango Sumba (Nairobi).

The IPDE was developed in the framework of the Joint Project on Diagnosis and Classification of Mental Disorders, Alcohol- and Drug-related Problems carried out by the WHO and US National Institutes of Health (formerly Alcohol, Drug and Mental Health Adminstration).

Manual

History of the IPDE

One of the aims of the World Health Organization (WHO) and US National Institutes of Health (NIH) joint program on psychiatric diagnosis and classification is the development and standardization of diagnostic assessment instruments for use in clinical research around the world.[1] The IPDE is a semistructured clinical interview developed within that program, and designed to assess the personality disorders in the ICD-10 and DSM-IV classification systems.

The IPDE is an outgrowth and modification for international use of the Personality Disorder Examination (PDE).[2] To facilitate the development of the IPDE, beginning in 1985 several workshops were convened. At these meetings representatives of the international psychiatric community discussed the format of the interview, the wording of items, and the development of a scoring manual. Translations were undertaken and frequent revisions made to reflect the experience of interviewers with trial versions. Finally, a field trial was undertaken in 1988 and 1989 at 14 participating centres in 11 countries in North America, Europe, Africa, and Asia.[3,4]

In August 1991 the principal investigators in the field trial met at WHO headquarters in Geneva to discuss the results and the experience of the interviewers with the IPDE. This resulted in some minor revisions of existing items. Subsequently additional modifications were made to accommodate the transition from DSM-III-R to DSM-IV. To offset concerns about the length of the interview, and to make it more acceptable to a wider range of clinicians and investigators, it was decided to issue the IPDE in modules. The complete interview would assess all of the disorders in both ICD-10 and DSM-IV. Separate modules would also be available for those who wished to limit the examination to one of the two classification systems.

ICD-10 and DSM-IV

DSM-IV[5] was designed for use in the US and is primarily the product of American psychiatric opinion. ICD-10[6] is intended for use throughout the world and reflects the views and needs of the international psychiatric community. The two are different but overlapping classification systems. There are slight differences in nomenclature: anankastic/obsessive-compulsive, anxious/avoidant, and dissocial/antisocial. In ICD-10, borderline and impulsive are viewed as subtypes of emotionally unstable, schizotypal is located with schizophrenia and delusional disorders, and narcissistic is not included. There are also some differences in the criteria required for various diagnoses. The IPDE field trial demonstrated that there was sufficient disagreement regarding the cases identified as personality disorders in DSM-III-R and ICD-10 to require the administration of the entire IPDE if one wished to make diagnoses in both systems.

Translations of the IPDE

Investigators at the various centres involved in the field trial have translated the instrument into the following languages: Dutch, French, German, Hindi, Japanese, Kannada, Norwegian, Swahili, and Tamil. Translations have also been made into other languages, including Danish, Estonian, Greek, Italian, Russian, and Spanish. Additional translations are contemplated. The translations were backtranslated into English by a psychiatrist or psychologist who had not seen the original English version. Variations and problems in the back-translation were then reviewed with those who undertook the original translation, and corrections were made when indicated.

Particular problems can arise when a semistructured interview like the IPDE is used with subjects who are illiterate and speak a regional or tribal dialect. Since written and spoken language are quite different in such populations, the interviewer must frequently depart from the literal text and improvise an equivalent question on the spot, in order to maintain communication with the subject. Although this is a potential source of error variance, the examiner's familiarity with the scope and meaning of the diagnostic criteria and with the intent of the original IPDE question, should keep such error within tolerable limits.

Structure of the IPDE

The IPDE is arranged in a format that attempts to provide the optimal balance between a spontaneous, natural clinical interview and the requirements of standardization and objectivity. At the beginning of the interview the subject is given the following instructions: 'The questions I am going to ask concern what you are like most of the time. I'm interested in what has been typical of you throughout your life, and not just recently. If you have changed and your answers might have been different at some time in the past, be sure to let me know.'

The questions flow in a natural sequence that is congenial to the clinician. They are arranged under six headings: work, self, interpersonal relationships, affects, reality testing, and impulse control. The headings are not only convenient labels, but they play an organizational or thematic role. At times the overlapping nature of the six domains required a somewhat arbitrary allocation of questions. For efficiency and convenience sometimes a question extends beyond the scope of the section where it appears. For example, many anankastic criteria are best assessed in the context of work functioning, but behaviour outside the realm of work is also considered, even though the questions appear in the 'Work' section of the interview.

The sections are usually introduced by open-ended inquiries that offer subjects an opportunity to discuss the topic as much as they choose. This helps to develop a set for the questions that follow, and provides a transition from the focus of the previous section. Although they are not scored as such, these introductory remarks of the subject provide a background against which to judge the clinical significance of some of the replies to the specific questions that follow. At times the comments also facilitate the task of the examiner in deciding whether to probe or pursue certain aspects of the subject's responses.

The criterion and its number, together with the name of the ICD-10 disorder, appear above the questions designed to assess it. Since the questions are merely an attempt to get at the criterion, this serves to remind the examiners what they are actually rating. Some criteria are followed by the designation *partial*, an indication that the item does not assess the entire criterion. This is done to preserve the topical focus of the interview. For example, it is more appropriate to inquire about an identity disorder in the sexual realm, when the subject of sex is being discussed, than to attempt to cover other manifestations of an identity disorder, such as uncertainty about values or career choice at the same point in the interview. There appears to be no consensus about exactly how long a behaviour should be present before it can be considered a personality trait. ICD-10 states that it should be stable and of long duration. Therefore, we have adopted the somewhat conservative convention that it should exist for a span of at least five years. Consideration was given to a three-year requirement, but it was decided that might too frequently lead to confounding episodic mental illnesses or responses to unusual or special life situations with the more enduring behaviour associated with personality. Some may feel this is too exacting, especially when applied to adolescents or young adults. Since users of the IPDE will differ in their predilection for making personality disorder diagnoses in adolescents, those who prefer a three-year requirement may adopt it for that age group. They should specify, however, that they have departed from the standard instructions. The use of anything less than a five-year time-frame with subjects over 20 years of age is discouraged.

ICD-10 dates the onset of the first manifestations of a personality disorder to late childhood or adolescence. For that reason we have taken the somewhat arbitrary position, that the requirements for at least one criterion of a disorder must have been fulfilled prior to age 25, before that particular disorder can be diagnosed. Age 25 years rather than an earlier age was selected to allow more informed and accurate judgements about many of the adult-oriented personality disorder criteria.

Clinical tradition notwithstanding, it is possible that personality transformations may occur in midlife or old age, and that a true personality disorder may emerge *de novo* at that time. In the absence of empirical data, rather than encourage premature closure on the subject, we have made provision in the IPDE for an optional *late onset* diagnosis. We have also provided the option of making a *past* diagnosis in someone who previously met the requirements, but has not done so during the past year (12 months).

Scope of the IPDE

The IPDE is not designed to survey the entire realm of personality. Its purpose is to identify those traits and behaviours that are relevant to an assessment of the criteria for personality disorders in the ICD-10 and DSM-IV classification systems. It neglects many neutral, positive, and adaptive traits, because they are irrelevant to a personality disorder assessment. It also does not cover other mental disorders, because there are instruments available for them. We recommend their use prior to the IPDE, to provide the examiner with clinical and historical information that is likely to enhance the reliability and validity of the questioning, probing, and scoring process. When it is not available from such an interview or from other sources, the IPDE examiner should obtain that information from the subject at the beginning of the interview (under 'Background information').

The IPDE ICD-10 Module examines every subject for the presence or absence of all the ICD-10 personality disorder criteria. It also provides a dimensional score for all subjects on each disorder, regardless of whether or not they fulfill the criteria for the disorder. This additional information supplements that based on categorical diagnosis alone. Because personality disorders often reflect the exaggerated presence of traits that are continuously distributed in the population at large, the dimensional scores are not only useful to the clinician, but they also provide the research investigator with greater reliability and more versatility in data analysis.

Appropriate subjects

The IPDE is not intended for subjects below the age of 18, although with slight modifications some investigators have found it useful with those as young as age 15. The interview is not appropriate for those with severe depression, psychosis, below-normal intelligence, or substantial cognitive impairment. Whether it should be used with patients in remission from a chronic psychotic illness is problematic. For example, can one distinguish residual schizophrenia or the interepisodic manifestations of manic-depression from a personality disorder? A number of investigators have found the IPDE useful in studies of those disorders, and the decision is left to the user.

Limitations of the IPDE

The IPDE is essentially a self-report instrument, and assumes that subjects are capable of providing valid descriptions of disturbances in their personality. However, individuals may be unaware of some of their traits. They may also be resistant to acknowledging behaviour, if it is socially undesirable or if its disclosure is likely to adversely affect what they believe to be their best interest. This is especially likely to occur in patients who wish to terminate treatment prematurely, or in those about to be discharged from a mental health facility. Others may exaggerate disturbances in their behaviour. This is sometimes observed in those who are frantically seeking help, or who are dissatisfied with their treatment or the amount of attention they are receiving. It may also be a reflection of certain personality traits. Although subjects may also feign traits or behaviour, particularly in compensation cases and some forensic and military situations, the IPDE discourages this by requiring documentation with convincing examples, anecdotes, and descriptions.

Patients in a dysphoric state may have a selective recall or distorted perception of some of their behaviour. They may also confuse normal and abnormal personality traits with the symptoms of a mental disorder. There is evidence[7] that the PDE was resistant to changes in the symptoms of anxiety and depression that occurred during the course of treatment, when those symptoms were of mild to moderate severity. This is not to imply that some clinical states, particularly those accompanied by severe symptoms, do not invalidate the assessment of personality. Additional research is required on this important subject. When possible, some investigators may wish to postpone the assessment until the symptoms of other mental disorders have remitted.

In ordinary clinical practice, a family member or close friend is often used as an additional source of information to offset the limitations of the self-report method. We have experimented with various procedures for augmenting the subject's responses on the IPDE with data from other sources. Failure to acknowledge a behaviour, particularly one that is especially frowned upon by others, is sometimes followed on the IPDE by such inquiries as, 'Have people told you that you're like that?' Affirmative replies are then pursued with the question, "Why do you think they've said that?" This approach can only be used selectively. If it were adopted in all situations where a behaviour has been denied, it would undermine the rapport between subject and examiner.

We have also tried a parallel form of the interview in which an informant was asked virtually the same questions about the patient. There were often discrepancies, and it was not always obvious who had provided the more valid information. It proved difficult to formulate a set of practical guidelines that stipulate the source that should be used in scoring a particular criterion. The problem is a complicated one, and a satisfactory resolution awaits the availability of more empirical data on the subject. Future studies may help identify those criteria that tend to produce discrepancies, and the characteristics of subjects and informants that might be used to determine the preferred source of information.

Meanwhile, we have adopted a practical, provisional solution to the informant problem. The IPDE has a second scoring column for informant data. If examiners have access to information from family, friends, mental health professionals, records, etc., that clearly contradicts a subject's responses regarding a particular criterion, then they may score the criterion in the informant column provided two requirements are met. Firstly, they should have more confidence in that information than they do in the subject; and secondly, the other source must satisfy the identical scoring guidelines that apply to the subject's response. Later, in entering ratings in the computer or transcribing them from the interview to the score-sheet, the scores based on the subject's report are bypassed in favour of those derived from the informant.

While it is necessary to administer the IPDE with knowledge of a subject's psychiatric history and current mental state, the examiner should avoid making detailed inquiries about the subject's personality prior to the interview. It is probably not advisable to confront subjects during the interview with discrepancies between their accounts and information obtained from others. Making them aware of the discrepancies could adversely affect rapport, and also create discord between the subject and informant.

Examiner qualifications and training

The IPDE ICD-10 Module presupposes a thorough familiarity with the ICD-10 classification system of mental disorders, and considerable training and experience in making psychiatric diagnoses. Like any semistructured clinical interview, its reliability and validity are inseparable from the qualifications and training of the person using it. It is designed for experienced psychiatrists, clinical psychologists, and those with comparable training, who are capable of making independent psychiatric diagnoses without a semistructured interview. It is not intended for use by clinicians in the early phase of their training, or by research assistants, nurses, and medical or graduate students.

The first step in training to use the IPDE is to study the interview and manual very thoroughly. Before the basics are mastered, the interview should be administered to several subjects primarily to get a 'feel' for it, and to make the instructions in this manual and the scoring guidelines more meaningful. Then the neophyte should examine a series of patients, following the instructions and scoring guidelines as closely as possible. This is best done with a colleague, someone who has already mastered the instrument or is also learning how to use it. These practice interviews should be followed by a critique, and a discussion of any problems in administration and scoring. Most clinicians will feel comfortable with the IPDE and have achieved a basic proficiency after having given about 10 interviews. As they examine more patients, they will find themselves making less use of the guides for questioning and scoring, but occasional reference to them is to be expected even by the seasoned examiner. We strongly recommend that those who wish to obtain the optimal training in the use of the IPDE, enroll in the course offered at one of the world-wide WHO training centres.

Administration of the IPDE

If the interview should take more than one to one and a half hours, there is danger that the examiner will not pursue responses with the same alertness and thoroughness, and that the subject's replies will become briefer and more perfunctory. In those circumstances the interview should be given on more than one occasion, if possible. However, interruptions in the middle of a section should be avoided.

The IPDE can only be administered properly when the examiner conducts an adequate clinical examination of the subject with appropriate probing to solicit examples, anecdotes, and additional details. This requires a thorough knowledge of the scope and meaning of each criterion and a correct application of the scoring guidelines. Ultimately, many of these become familiar to examiners, and there is no need to constantly refer to them during the interview.

Initial replies of the subject that suggest a positive rating are rarely sufficient for scoring a criterion. They must be supplemented and supported by convincing descriptions or examples. Examiners must use their clinical judgement to determine the length of the descriptions and the number of examples that are required. When in doubt, they should always ask for more rather than less. However, they should avoid 'leading the witness,' or being influenced by a 'halo' effect. For example, if the subject has already met three of the required four criteria for a diagnosis, the examples regarding a possible fourth criterion should not be viewed any differently than if the subject had previously not met any criterion. Interviewers should not hesitate to tactfully inquire about apparent contradictions in responses. Although the examiners should score the interview as they go along, they should correct the scoring of an earlier item, when subsequent information elicited during the interview requires it. Recording the subject's responses verbatim is not required, but it can provide a permanent record of a considerable amount of useful information, that is not conveyed by diagnoses or dimensional scores alone.

Scoring conventions

Much of the behaviour described in the ICD-10 personality disorder criteria exists on a continuum with normality. The IPDE scoring is based on the convention that a behaviour or trait may be absent or normal (0), exaggerated or accentuated (1), and criterion level or pathological (2). A few items are not applicable to some subjects, and they are scored 'NA'. The '?' scoring category is reserved for occasions when subjects, despite encouragement, refuse to answer a question or state that they are unable to do so. It is not used to designate uncertainty on the part of the examiner about rating the item.

Duration

If the behaviour or trait has not been present for a timespan of at least five years it does not receive a positive score, even though it meets all the requirements concerning frequency, intensity, subjective distress, and social or occupational impairment. A positive score (except 'past') is also *not* given when the behaviour has not occurred at all during the past year (12 months). The only exceptions to the past year (12 months) rule are those behaviours that occur relatively infrequently, yet have considerable clinical significance. Those items (10, 15, 26, 34, 55, 59, 60, 61) are designated by an asterisk next to the item number on the interview schedule. However, they too must have occurred *at least once during the past five years* to receive a positive score. Otherwise, like other items that meet all the requirements except past year (12 months), they should be scored 'past'.

Age at onset

The IPDE requires that behaviour indicative of at least one criterion of a personality disorder be present prior to age 25, before that particular disorder can be diagnosed. The remaining criteria for the disorder may become evident after age 25, provided the requirement of five years duration is met. This rule exists for each individual disorder. However, when a subject meets all the requirements for a diagnosis except that regarding onset by age 25, an optional diagnosis may be recorded with the designation, 'late onset'.

Timeframe and age at onset probes

The examiner must use a predetermined set of probes to determine whether a subject has met the duration and age at onset requirements. The probes may be selected to fit the particular responses and criteria, and may be varied to avoid monotony or stereotypy. Ordinarily examiners should devise their own probes only when the subject does not provide adequate replies to the recommended ones. It is *not* necessary to ask subjects whether the behaviour has occurred during the past year. The assumption is that it has or they would either not have reported it, or noted that a change had taken place, since they are reminded to do so several times during the course of the interview. Of course, if examiners have reason to doubt that it has occurred during the past year, then they should question the subject about it.

Duration and age at onset probes

- How long have you been like that?
- How long has that been going on?
- How long have you been that way?
- When did that start?
- How old were you when that began?
- At what age did that start?
- Have you been that way for a long time?

Frequency

Scoring usually requires a knowledge of the frequency with which the subject manifests the behaviour, because it is often one of the grounds for distinguishing scores of '0', '1', '2'. Some IPDE questions contain frequency information, e.g., 'Do you often change from your usual mood to feeling very irritable, etc.?' This should *not* be relied upon to establish the actual frequency. Replies acknowledging the presence of the behaviour associated with the criterion require that the examiner ask how often it occurs by using one of the predetermined frequency probes. The sole exception is when subjects spontaneously supply the frequency in their replies.

Frequency probes

- How often are you like that?
- How often does that happen?
- How often do you behave like that?

Recording the scores

Required scoring

Immediately after questioning the subject about a particular item, the examiner records the score in the *first* column. The second column is never used during the interview itself. It is reserved for information from informants or records, when it is discrepant with the interview data, and the rater has more confidence in that than in the subject. The information, however, is subject to the same scoring guidelines as the subject's responses.

If the subject does not meet the requirements stipulated in the manual for a positive score (1 or 2), the rater places a circle around '0'. If the subject meets all the requirements for a positive score (1 or 2), including onset prior to age 25, the rater *circles* the appropriate number (1 or 2). If the subject meets all the requirements for a positive score except age at onset, the rater *underlines* the appropriate number (1 or 2). If subjects insist they are unable to answer a question or refuse to do so, the rater places a circle around '?'. If the criterion does not apply to the subject, the rater places a circle around 'NA'.

Optional scoring

If examiners wish to record a personality disorder that was present in the past, but no longer exists, they must use an additional set of scoring notations in certain very specific situations. If a subject meets all the requirements for a positive score, including that of five years duration and age at onset before 25, but has not displayed the behaviour at all during the past year (12 months), the rater should place an 'X' through the appropriate number (1 or 2). If a subject meets all the requirements for a positive score, including that of five years duration, except that onset has occurred after age 25, and the behaviour has not been present at all during the past year (12 months), the rater should underline the 'X'. It is important to remember that asterisked items (10, 15, 26, 34, 55, 59, 60, 61) are exempt from the requirement that they occur during the past 12 months. Therefore, those *exempt* items should be scored 'past' only when they occurred prior to but not during the past five years; otherwise they satisfy the requirements for a current disorder.

Computer scoring

The IPDE diagnoses and dimensional scores are determined after the completion of the interview. The most efficient method is to use the computer scoring program*. The scores from the interview schedule or answer sheet are entered directly into a personal computer. The program is written with operator prompts, and the user responds to questions regarding the task to be performed and the management of the data, which may be sent to a printer and saved in a disk file. The entire procedure takes approximately 10 minutes.

The printout provides the following information for each ICD-10 disorder: criteria present or absent; number of criteria met; diagnosis – definite, probable (one criterion less than the required number), negative, late onset (optional), past (optional); dimensional score; and number of criteria based on informants. The criteria met by the subject are also printed verbatim.

The IPDE program will execute properly under either the BASICA program supplied with IBM PCs or GWBASIC supplied with MS-DOS, PC compatible systems, and requires a 2.0 or greater version of DOS. It is supplied on a single 360K diskette with accompanying software. The diskette also has a short batch file for installation on a hard disk drive.

Handscoring

The IPDE may also be handscored by clerical personnel. All of the scores are transcribed onto summary scoresheets that contain step-by-step algorithmic directions.

Frequently asked questions about the administration of the IPDE

Q. Do I ask every subject all of the questions on the IPDE?

A. Ask every question that is flush with the left-hand margin unless directed otherwise. Indented questions preceded by 'If Yes' or 'If No' are asked if the subject provides the appropriate response. When an indented question is asked, be sure to include any subsequent questions that are aligned with it.

Q. Should the questions be asked verbatim?

A. Yes. Do not change the wording or embellish the question with your own comments, a common error of beginners.

---

* The IPDE Computer Scoring Program for ICD-10 Diagnoses can be obtained from the Division of Mental Health and Prevention of Substance Abuse, World Health Organization, CH-1211 Geneva 27, Switzerland.

Q. What do you do when subjects misunderstand a question or say that they do not understand it?

A. Rephrase the question in your own words, so that you approximate the intent of the original question. In doing so be mindful of the criterion assessed by the question.

Q. Is it necessary to ask a question, if the subject has already provided the answer in response to a previous question?

A. *Never* assume that you know the answer, because of a response to a similar or related question. However, if the subject has already provided sufficient information, so that nothing would be gained from asking the question, and you are confident about scoring it, then it need not be asked. If you require more information or additional details, ask the question with an allusion to the subject's previous reference to it.

Q. Do you score the subject's report, or base the score on your clinical impression?

A. Score the report, except in those rare instances when directed otherwise. If the response appears to contradict a previous comment, ask the subject to explain the apparent contradiction.

Q. Suppose the subject's behaviour during the interview seems to contradict the reply to a question? For example, the subject reports that he or she is rarely angry, yet displays obvious anger during the interview.

A. Ask the subject to reconcile the apparent contradiction. This may lead to a revision of the previous response. If it does not, then score the response and not the behaviour during the interview. Remember, the latter may not be representative of the way the subject has been during the previous five years, particularly if he or she is currently in a dysphoric mental state. Of course, informant information is particularly useful in situations like this.

Q. At the end of the interview several criteria are rated entirely on the basis of the subject's behaviour during the interview. Isn't this inconsistent with the use of a five-year timeframe in the remainder of the interview?

A. Those criteria cannot be adequately assessed by self-report. Admittedly the features could be present during the interview without necessarily being characteristic of the subject. They also may not surface during the interview, yet be evident at other times. There is no other practical way of judging the presence or absence of these particular criteria, except to rely on informant information.

Q. What about the criteria that are exempt from the 'past year' (12 months) requirement?

A. The behaviour must have occurred *at least once during the last five years*. If it only occurred prior to the last five years, those employing the optional scoring for a 'past' personality disorder would score it positively, using the appropriate notation.

Q. If I elect to score a criterion as 'past', must I determine whether it overlaps in time with the other criteria that are scored positively for that disorder?

A. No. That would make the scoring too unwieldy, because the examiner would have to note the timeframe next to all positive ratings. The subject might also have difficulty recalling whether the behaviour associated with the various criteria overlapped in time.

Q. Affirmative answers to questions that take the form, 'Have people told you that you're like that?,' are followed by, 'Why do you think they've said that?' How should replies to these follow-up questions be handled?

A. Request examples, anecdotes, and descriptions. After any necessary probing, score the item according to the usual guidelines.

Q. What if subjects endorse a trait or behaviour, but say that they are unable to provide examples?

A. If despite encouragement they persist in saying so, then a positive score should not be given. This will result in occasional false-negative ratings, but experience suggests that to deviate from the rule would probably lead to an unacceptable number of false-positive ratings. If subjects really have the trait to a clinically meaningful degree, they should be able to provide anecdotes or examples.

Abbreviating the IPDE

This module of the IPDE is designed to assess all of the personality disorders in ICD-10, and the interview should be administered in its entirety whenever possible. Because of time constraints some users may be unable to give the complete interview to all subjects; others may be interested in only certain specific disorders. In those situations two options are available.

The first option is to omit the items that do not pertain to the disorders of interest. In doing so, however, the examiner should always be sure to include the introductory, open-ended questions at the beginning of each section, if there are questions in that section that pertain to the disorders that are being assessed.

The second option is to use the self-administered 'IPDE Screening Questionnaire' to eliminate subjects who are unlikely to have a personality disorder or the particular disorders of interest. The screen is expected to produce a considerable number of false-positive but relatively few false-negative cases *vis-à-vis* the interview. The rates of case misidentification, however, are likely to vary considerably depending on the base-rates of the disorders in the population in which it is employed.

It is especially important to recognize that personality disorder questionnaires and semistructured clinical interviews are not interchangeable.[8] Therefore, under no circumstances should the 'IPDE Screening Questionnaire' be used to make a psychiatric diagnosis. Nor should it be used to calculate dimensional scores, with the expectation that they will be equivalent to those based on the IPDE itself.

Reliability and validity of the IPDE

The interrater agreement and temporal stability of the IPDE were studied at 14 clinical facilities in 11 countries in North America, Europe, Africa, and Asia. The field trial employed 58 psychiatrists and clinical psychologists as interviewers and observers of 716 patients. The reliability and stability of the IPDE were roughly similar to what has been reported with instruments used to diagnose the psychoses, mood, anxiety, and substance use disorders.[4]

Establishing the validity of semistructured clinical interviews has proved to be a more elusive undertaking, because of the absence of an acceptable gold standard. The use of clinical consensus as that standard is problematic without information about the reliability and validity of the clinicians themselves. The advantage of semistructured interviews like the IPDE, is that they have a certain procedural validity that makes their conclusions more readily exportable, and less susceptible to institutional and regional biases. In theory, they provide clinicians and investigators with a more uniform method of case identification, and thus facilitate the comparison and replication of research findings. It was the opinion of most of the clinicians who participated in the field trial, that the IPDE was a useful and essentially valid method of assessing personality disorders for research purposes.

References

1   Jablensky, A., Sartorius, N., Hirschfeld. R. & Pardes, H. Diagnosis and classification of mental disorders and alcohol- and drug-related problems: A research agenda for the 1980s. *Psychological Medicine*, 1983;**13**:907–21.

2   Loranger, A.W. *Personality Disorder Examination (PDE) Manual.* Yonkers: DV Communications, 1988.

3   Loranger, A.W., Hirschfeld, R.M.A., Sartorius, N. & Regier, D.A. The WHO/ADAMHA International Pilot Study of Personality Disorders: Background and purpose. *Journal of Personality Disorders*, 1991;**5**:296–306.

4   Loranger, A.W., Sartorius, N., Andreoli, A., Berger, P., Buchheim, P., Channabasavanna, S.M., Coid, B., Dahl, A., Diekstra, R.F.W., Ferguson, B., Jacobsberg, L.B., Mombour, W., Pull, C., Ono, Y. & Regier, D.A. The World Health Organization/Alcohol, Drug Abuse, and Mental Health Administration International Pilot Study of Personality Disorders. *Archives of General Psychiatry*, 1994;**51**:215–24.

5   American Psychiatric Association, Committee on Nomenclature and Statistics. *Diagnostic and Statistical Manual of Mental Disorders, revised 4th edn.* Washington DC: American Psychiatric Press, 1994.

6   World Health Organization. *The ICD-10 Classification of Mental and Behavioural Disorders: Diagnostic Criteria for Research.* Geneva: World Health Organization, 1993.

7   Loranger, A.W., Lenzenweger, M.F., Gartner, A.F., Lehmann Susman, V., Herzig, J., Zammit, G.K., Gartner, J.D., Abrams, R.C. & Young, R.C. Trait-state artifacts and the diagnosis of personality disorders. *Archives of General Psychiatry*, 1991;**48**:720–8.

8   Loranger, A.W. Are current self-report and interview measures adequate for epidemiological studies of personality disorders? *Journal of Personality Disorders*, 1992;**6**:313–25.

ICD-10 criteria and corresponding IPDE items

F60.0   **Paranoid personality disorder**

At least four of the following must be present:

(1)   excessive sensitivity to setbacks and rebuffs **38**
(2)   tendency to bear grudges persistently, e.g. refusal to forgive insults, injuries, or slights **34**
(3)   suspiciousness and a pervasive tendency to distort experience by misconstruing the neutral or friendly actions of others as hostile or contemptuous **35**
(4)   a combative and tenacious sense of personal rights out of keeping with the actual situation **31**
(5)   recurrent suspicions, without justification, regarding sexual fidelity of spouse or sexual partner **55**
(6)   persistent self-referential attitude, associated particularly with excessive self-importance **36**
(7)   preoccupation with unsubstantiated "conspiratorial" explanations of events either immediate to the patient or in the world at large **57**

F60.1   **Schizoid personality disorder**

At least four of the following criteria must be present:

(1)   few, if any, activities provide pleasure **42**
(2)   display of emotional coldness, detachment, or flattened affectivity **67**
(3)   limited capacity to express either warm, tender feelings or anger toward others **39, 44**
(4)   an appearance of indifference to either praise or criticism **37**
(5)   little interest in having sexual experiences with another person (taking into account age) **53**
(6)   consistent choice of solitary activities **22**
(7)   excessive preoccupation with fantasy and introspection **18**
(8)   no desire for, or possession of, any close friends or confiding relationships (or only one) **19**
(9)   marked insensitivity to prevailing social norms and conventions; disregard for such norms and conventions is unintentional **66**

F60.2   **Dissocial personality disorder**

At least three of the following must be present:

(1)   callous unconcern for the feelings of others **29**
(2)   gross and persistent attitude of irresponsibility and disregard for social norms, rules, and obligations **61**

(3)   incapacity to maintain enduring relationships, though with no difficulty in establishing them **20**

(4)   very low tolerance to frustration and a low threshold for discharge of aggression, including violence **15, 60**

(5)   incapacity to experience guilt, or to profit from adverse experience, particularly punishment **62, 64**

(6)   marked proneness to blame others, or to offer plausible rationalizations for the behaviour that has brought the individual into conflict with society **63**

F60.3   Emotionally unstable personality disorder

F60.30   Impulsive type

At least three of the following must be present, one of which must be (2):

(1)   marked tendency to act unexpectedly and without consideration of the consequences **58**

(2)   marked tendency to quarrelsome behaviour and to conflicts with others, especially when impulsive acts are thwarted or criticized **30**

(3)   liability to outbursts of anger or violence, with inability to control the resulting behavioural explosions **43**

(4)   difficulty in maintaining any course of action that offers no immediate reward **11**

(5)   unstable and capricious mood **50**

F60.31   Borderline type

At least three of the symptoms mentioned in Impulsive type (F60.30) must be present, with at least two of the following in addition:

(1)   disturbances in and uncertainty about self-image, aims, and internal preferences (including sexual) **5, 6, 7, 25, 56**

(2)   liability to become involved in intense and unstable relationships, often leading to emotional crises **26**

(3)   excessive efforts to avoid abandonment **48**

(4)   recurrent threats or acts of self-harm **59**

(5)   chronic feelings of emptiness **45**

F60.4   Histrionic personality disorders

At least four of the following must be present:

(1)   self-dramatization, theatricality, or exaggerated expression of emotions **40**

(2)   suggestibility (the individual is easily influenced by others or by circumstances) **12**

(3)   shallow and labile affectivity **49**

(4)   continual seeking for excitement and activities in which the individual is the centre of attention **16, 41**

(5)   inappropriate seductiveness in appearance or behaviour **54**
(6)   over-concern with physical attractiveness **17**

F60.5   Anankastic personality disorder

Note: This disorder is often referred to as obsessive-compulsive personality disorder.
At least four of the following must be present:

(1)   feelings of excessive doubt and caution **9**
(2)   preoccupation with details, rules, lists, order, organization, or schedule **3**
(3)   perfectionism that interferes with task completion **2**
(4)   excessive conscientiousness and scrupulousness **14**
(5)   undue preoccupation with productivity to the exclusion of pleasure and interpersonal relationships **1**
(6)   excessive pedantry and adherence to social conventions **65**
(7)   rigidity and stubbornness **28**
(8)   unreasonable insistence by the individual that others submit to exactly his or her way of doing things, or unreasonable reluctance to allow others to do things **27**

F60.6   Anxious [avoidant] personality disorder

At least four of the following must be present:

(1)   persistent and pervasive feelings of tension and apprehension **52**
(2)   belief that one is socially inept, personally unappealing, or inferior to others **13**
(3)   excessive preoccupation with being criticized or rejected in social situations **24**
(4)   unwillingness to become involved with people unless certain of being liked **23**
(5)   restrictions in lifestyle because of need for physical security **51**
(6)   avoidance of social or occupational activities that involve significant interpersonal contact, because of fear of criticism, disapproval, or rejection **4, 21**

F60.7   Dependent personality disorder

At least four of the following must be present:

(1)   encouraging or allowing others to make most of one's important life decisions **10**
(2)   subordination of one's own needs to those of others on whom one is dependent, and undue compliance with their wishes **33**
(3)   unwillingness to make even reasonable demands on the people one depends on **32**
(4)   feeling uncomfortable or helpless when alone, because of exaggerated fears of inability to care for oneself **46**

(5) preoccupation with fears of being left to care for oneself **47**

(6) limited capacity to make everyday decisions without an excessive amount of advice and reassurance from others **8**

F60.9   **Personality disorder unspecified**

The IPDE assigns this diagnosis (definite) when someone fulfills 10 or more criteria from the various personality disorders, but does not meet the requirements for the diagnosis (definite) of any specific disorder. It assigns this diagnosis (probable) when someone fulfills 9 criteria from the various personality disorders, but does not meet the requirements for the diagnosis (definite or probable) of any specific disorder.

IPDE ICD-10 module screening questionnaire

Last Name	First Name	Middle I.	Date

Directions

1 The purpose of this questionnaire is to learn what type of person you have been during the **past five years**.

2 Please do not skip any items. If you are not sure of an answer, select the one-TRUE or FALSE-which is **more likely** to be correct. There is no time limit, but do not spend too much time thinking about the answer to any single statement.

3 When the answer is TRUE, **circle** the letter T. When the answer is FALSE, **circle** the letter F.

1	I usually get fun and enjoyment out of life.	T	F
2	I don't react well when someone offends me.	T	F
3	I'm not fussy about little details.	T	F
4	I can't decide what kind of person I want to be.	T	F
5	I show my feelings for everyone to see.	T	F
6	I let others make my big decisions for me.	T	F
7	I usually feel tense or nervous.	T	F
8	I almost never get angry about anything.	T	F
9	I go to extremes to try to keep people from leaving me.	T	F
10	I'm a very cautious person.	T	F
11	I've never been arrested.	T	F
12	People think I'm cold and detached.	T	F
13	I get into very intense relationships that don't last.	T	F
14	Most people are fair and honest with me.	T	F
15	I find it hard to disagree with people if I depend on them a lot.	T	F
16	I feel awkward or out of place in social situations.	T	F
17	I'm too easily influenced by what goes on around me.	T	F
18	I usually feel bad when I hurt or mistreat someone.	T	F
19	I argue or fight when people try to stop me from doing what I want.	T	F
20	At times I've refused to hold a job, even when I was expected to.	T	F
21	When I'm praised or criticized I don't show others my reaction.	T	F
22	I've held grudges against people for years.	T	F
23	I spend too much time trying to do things perfectly.	T	F
24	People often make fun of me behind my back.	T	F
25	I've never threatened suicide or injured myself on purpose.	T	F
26	My feelings are like the weather; they're always changing.	T	F
27	I fight for my rights even when it annoys people.	T	F
28	I like to dress so I stand out in a crowd.	T	F
29	I will lie or con someone if it serves my purpose.	T	F
30	I don't stick with a plan if I don't get results right away.	T	F
31	I have little or no desire to have sex with anyone.	T	F
32	People think I'm too strict about rules and regulations.	T	F
33	I usually feel uncomfortable or helpless when I'm alone.	T	F
34	I won't get involved with people until I'm certain they like me.	T	F
35	I would rather not be the centre of attention.	T	F
36	I think my spouse (or lover) may be unfaithful to me.	T	F
37	Sometimes I get so angry I break or smash things.	T	F
38	I've had close friendships that lasted a long time.	T	F
39	I worry a lot that people may not like me.	T	F
40	I often feel "empty" inside.	T	F
41	I work so hard I don't have time left for anything else.	T	F
42	I worry about being left alone and having to care for myself.	T	F
43	A lot of things seem dangerous to me that don't bother most people.	T	F
44	I have a reputation for being a flirt.	T	F
45	I don't ask favors from people I depend on a lot.	T	F
46	I prefer activities that I can do by myself.	T	F

47	I lose my temper and get into physical fights.	T	F
48	People think I'm too stiff or formal.	T	F
49	I often seek advice or reassurance about everyday decisions.	T	F
50	I keep to myself even when there are other people around.	T	F
51	It's hard for me to stay out of trouble.	T	F
52	I'm convinced there's a conspiracy behind many things in the world.	T	F
53	I'm very moody.	T	F
54	It's hard for me to get used to a new way of doing things.	T	F
55	Most people think I'm a strange person.	T	F
56	I take chances and do reckless things.	T	F
57	Everyone needs a friend or two to be happy.	T	F
58	I'm more interested in my own thoughts than what goes on around me.	T	F
59	I usually try to get people to do things my way.	T	F

IPDE ICD-10 module screening questionnaire scoring summary

Last Name	First Name	Middle I.	Date

1 Circle the item numbers not followed by F, if they were answered True.
2 Circle the remaining item numbers (those followed by F), if they were answered False.
3 If three or more items from a disorder are circled, the subject has failed the screen for that disorder, and should be interviewed. Clinicians and investigators may wish to adopt lower or higher screening standards, depending on the nature of the sample, and the relative   importance to them of errors of sensitivity (false-negative cases) vs. specificity (false-positive cases). The screen should not be used to make a diagnosis or to calculate a dimensional score for a personality disorder.

F60.0	Paranoid:	2	14F	22	24	27	36	52		
F60.1	Schizoid:	1F	8	12	21	31	46	55	57F	58
F60.2	Dissocial:	11F	18F	20	29	38F	47	51		
F60.30	Impulsive:	19	30	37	53	56				
F60.31	Borderline:	4	9	13	25F	40				
F60.4	Histrionic:	5	17	26	28	35F	44			
F60.5	Anankastic:	3F	10	23	32	41	48	54	59	
F60.6	Anxious:	7	16	34	39	43	50			
F60.7	Dependent:	6	15	33	42	45	49			

IPDE ICD-10 module* interview schedule

Last Name   First Name   Middle I.   Sex: M F

Examiner   Date(s)   Time Required for Interview

Background information
Optional if already known

How old are you?

Are you married?
  If no: Were you ever married?

Do you have any children?

Are your parents living?
  If yes: How old are they?
  If no: When did they die?

Do you have brothers or sisters?
  If yes: How old are they?

With whom do you live?

How far along did you go in school?

At what age did you finish school?

What is your occupation?

Have you had other occupations during your life?
  If yes: What?

Tell me briefly why you are /here/in the hospital/in treatment/.

Have you ever sought professional help for personal problems or a mental disorder at any (other) time in your life?
  If yes: Tell me about it.

---

*   Copies of the IPDE ICD-10 Module can be obtained from the Division of Mental Health and Prevention of Substance Abuse, World Health Organization, CH-1211 Geneva 27, Switzerland.

The questions I am going to ask concern what you are like most of the time. I'm interested in what has been typical of you throughout your life and not just recently. If you have changed and your answers might have been different at some time in the past, be sure to let me know.

I. Work

If the subject has rarely or never worked, and is not a housewife/home-maker, student, or recent graduate, circle NA for 1 and proceed to 2.

I would like to begin by discussing your life at work (school). How well do you usually function in your work (at school)?

What annoyances or problems keep occurring in your work (at school)?

---

1.   0   1   2   ?   NA   **0   1   2**
Undue preoccupation with productivity to the exclusion of pleasure and interpersonal relationships
Anankastic: 5

Do you spend so much time working that you don't have time left for anything else?
If yes: Tell me about it.

Do you spend so much time working that you (also) neglect other people?
If yes: Tell me about it.

The examiner should be alert to the use of rationalizations to defend the behaviour. The fact that work itself may be pleasurable to the subject should not influence the scoring. There is no requirement that the subject actually enjoy the work, although that is often the case. Personal ambition, high economic aspirations, or inefficient use of time, are also unacceptable excuses. Exoneration due to economic necessity should be extended only when supported by convincing explanations. Allowance should be made for short-term, unusual circumstances, e.g., physicians in training who have little or no control over their work schedule. Avoidance of interpersonal relationships or leisure activities for reasons other than devotion to work is not within the scope of the criterion.

2   Undue preoccupation with work that usually prevents any significant pursuit of both leisure activities and interpersonal relationships.

1   Undue preoccupation with work that occasionally prevents any significant pursuit of both leisure activities and interpersonal relationships.

     Undue preoccupation with work that usually prevents any significant pursuit of either leisure activities or interpersonal relationships but not both.

0   Denied or rarely or never leads to exclusion of leisure activities or interpersonal relationships.

---

2.   0   1   2   ?   **0   1   2**
Perfectionism that interferes with task completion
Anankastic: 3

Are you more of a perfectionist than almost anyone you know?

If yes: Does it slow you down a lot or prevent you from getting things done on time?

   If yes: Tell me about it.

Many subjects view themselves as perfectionistic, but do not have the trait to a pronounced degree or to the extent that it significantly interferes with their functioning. It is particularly important to verify that there is an effect on task completion or productivity.

2   Perfectionism frequently prevents the completion of work, or interferes with productivity.

1   Perfectionism occasionally prevents the completion of work, or interferes with productivity.

0   Denied, rarely or never prevents the completion of work, or interferes with productivity.

3.   0   1   2   ?   **0   1   2**
Preoccupation with details, rules, lists, order, organization, or schedule
Anankastic: 2

Are you fussy about little details?
If yes: Do you spend much more time on them than you really have to?
  If yes: Does that prevent you from getting as much work done as you're expected to do?

  If yes: Tell me about it.

Do you spend so much time scheduling or organizing things that you don't have time left to do the job you're really supposed to do?
If yes: Tell me about it.

The subject is so concerned with the method or details of accomplishing a task or objective, that they almost become an end in themselves, consuming much more time and effort than is necessary, and thereby preventing the task from being accomplished, or markedly prolonging the time required to achieve the objective. The subject need not display all of the features enumerated in the criterion.

2   Convincing evidence supported by examples that the behaviour frequently interferes with reasonable expectations of productivity.

1   Convincing evidence supported by examples that the behaviour occasionally interferes with reasonable expectations of productivity.

0   Denied, rare, or the consequences are insignificant.

4.   0   1   2   ?   NA   **0**   **1**   **2**

Avoidance of occupational activities that involve significant interpersonal contact, because of fear of criticism, disapproval, or rejection

Anxious [avoidant]:   6 (partial)

Do you usually try to avoid jobs or things you have to do at work(school), that bring you into contact with other people?

If yes: Give me some examples.

Why do you think you do that?

The criterion is not so readily applicable to housewives/homemakers and ordinarily should be scored NA with them. They have an opportunity to qualify on the other half of the criterion (**21**, avoidance of social activities). "Significant interpersonal contact" in this context means that the subject would likely be engaged in conversation with others. It does not refer to the mere physical presence of others in the same building or work area. The reason for the avoidance must be fear of criticism, disapproval or rejection.

2   Almost always avoids jobs or work(school) assignments that involve significant interpersonal contact. Subject provides one or more of these as the primary reason: fear of criticism, disapproval or rejection.

1   Often avoids jobs or work(school) assignments that involve significant interpersonal contact. Subject provides one or more of these as the primary reason: fear of criticism, disapproval or rejection.

Almost always avoids jobs or work(school) assignments that involve significant interpersonal contact. Subject acknowledges one or more of the three reasons, but insists that they are not the primary reason.

0   Denied, infrequent, not supported by convincing examples, or avoidance is due to other reasons.

II. SELF

Now let me ask some questions about the kind of person you are.

How would you describe your personality?

Have you always been like that?
If no: When did you change?
  What were you like before?

---

5.   0   1   2   ?   **0**   **1**   **2**
Disturbances in and uncertainty about self-image
Emotionally unstable; Borderline type: 1 (partial)

Do you think one of your problems is that you're not sure what kind of person you are?
If yes: How does that affect your life?

Do you behave as though you don't know what to expect of yourself?
If yes: Are you so different with different people or in different situations that you don't behave like the same person?
  If yes: Give me some examples.

  If no: Have others told you that you're like that?
    If yes: Why do you think they've said that?

In this context "uncertainty about self-image" may manifest itself in different ways, any one of which, if obviously present, is sufficient for a positive score. Subjects may be uncertain about what kind of person they are, because their behaviour is so different at various times or with different people, that they do not know what to expect of themself. Their behaviour may be inconsistent, erratic, or contradictory. Or they may be chameleon-like and take on the identity or personality of the particular person they are with at the moment. It is not necessary that subjects acknowledge or be aware that this is the source of distress or problems. Strikingly different behaviour or views of oneself confined to discrete episodes of illness are not within the scope of the criterion. However, changes in self-image or erratic behaviour indicative of an inconsistent sense of self, may be counted when they occur in conjunction with chronic anxiety or chronic depression.

2   Obvious and well documented persistent uncertainty about self-image, as described above.

1   Probable but less well documented persistent uncertainty about self-image, as described above.

0   Absent, doubtful, or not well supported by examples.

---

6.   0   1   2   ?   **0   1   2**
Disturbances in and uncertainty about aims
Emotionally unstable; Borderline type: 1 (partial)

What would you like to accomplish during your life?

Do your ideas about this change often?
If yes: Tell me about it.

**Not asked of housewives/homemakers, adolescents, students, and those who have
never or almost never worked.**
Do you often wonder whether you've made the right choice of job or career?
If yes: How does that affect you?

Asked only of housewives/homemakers.
Do you often wonder whether you've made the right choice in becoming a housewife/home-
maker?
If yes: How does that affect you?

Adolescents, students, and those who have never or almost never worked.
Have you made up your mind about what kind of job or career you would like to have?
If no: How does that affect you?

> The requirements for this criterion may be fulfilled in any one of several dif-
> ferent ways. Subjects may report that they cannot decide about their
> long-term goals or career choice, and that this has an obvious effect on the
> way they lead their life. They may deny that they are uncertain about them,
> but it may be obvious from their behaviour, which is characterized by persis-
> tently erratic or fluctuating consideration or selection of strikingly different
> careers or long-term goals. Persons 30 years of age or older who have not
> embarked on a career path (when one is available to them), or insist that they
> have no idea at all about what their long-term goals are, should receive a
> score of 2. The criterion should be scored conservatively with adolescents and
> not usually given to them.

2   Obvious and well documented persistent uncertainty about long-term goals
    or career choice.

1   Probable but less well documented or persistent uncertainty about long-term
    goals or career choice.

0   Absent, doubtful, or not supported by convincing examples.

7.   0   1   2   ?   **0**   **1**   **2**
Disturbances in and uncertainty about internal preferences
Emotionally unstable; Borderline type: 1 (partial)

Do you have trouble deciding what's important in life?
If yes: How does that affect you or the way you live your life?

Do you have trouble deciding what's morally right and wrong?
If yes: How does that affect you or the way you live your life?

In this context "internal preferences" refers both to issues of ethics and morality ("right and wrong") and to values (what is important in life). For a positive score both are not required. Subjects may qualify for either in two ways. They may report that they are so uncertain about internal preferences, that it causes subjective distress or problems in social or occupational functioning. Or they may, with or without acknowledgment or awareness of any uncertainty, demonstrate the phenomenon by extremely erratic or inconsistent behaviour indicative of uncertain values.

2   Obvious and well documented persistent uncertainty about internal preferences as described above.

1   Probable but less well documented or persistent uncertainty about internal preferences as described above.

0   Absent, doubtful, or not well supported by examples.

8.   0   1   2   ?   **0   1   2**
Limited capacity to make everyday decisions without an excessive amount of advice and reassurance from others
Dependent: 6

Are you usually able to make ordinary, everyday decisions without asking others for advice or reassurance?
If no: Give me some examples.

Indecisiveness not associated with the need for advice or reassurance is not within the scope of the criterion, which concerns ordinary, everyday, types of decisions, and is not meant to include unusual, special, or major decisions. The essence of the criterion is the inability to make these ordinary decisions without seeking advice or confirmation from others. Both elements, advice and reassurance, are not required.

2   Frequently depends on others for an excessive amount of advice or reassurance before making decisions about ordinary matters, so that the decisions are not otherwise made.

1   Occasionally depends on others for an excessive amount of advice or reassurance before making decisions about ordinary matters, so that the decisions are not otherwise made.

0   Denied, rare, or examples not convincing.

---

9.   0   1   2   ?   **0**   **1**   **2**
Feelings of excessive doubt and caution
Anankastic: 1

Do you have a lot of doubts about things?
If yes: Does that upset you or cause any problems for you?
  If yes: Tell me about it.

Are you very cautious and afraid of making a mistake?
If yes: Does that bother you or cause any problems for you?
  If yes: Give me some examples of what you mean.

If the preceding item (**8**) was scored 1 or 2, the subject should be questioned carefully to establish that the reason for the excessive doubt is not solely the dependent's need for advice and reassurance from others. Caution is reflected by exceptional concern about making a mistake. Caution limited to concerns about physical security is not within the scope of the criterion. For a 2 score there must be evidence of both doubt and caution, and indications that they are sometimes a source of distress or problems.

2   Frequently shows excessive doubt **and** caution, and this sometimes causes distress or problems in social or occupational functioning.

1   Frequently shows excessive doubt **or** caution, but not both, and this sometimes causes distress or problems in social or occupational functioning.

Occasionally shows excessive doubt **and** caution, and this sometimes causes distress or problems in social or occupational functioning.

0   Denied, rare, or examples unconvincing.

*10.   0   1   2   ?   **0   1   2**
            Encouraging or allowing others to make most of one's important life
            decisions
            Dependent: 1

Do you let other people take charge of your life for you?
If yes: Tell me about it.

Do you let them make your important decisions for you?
If yes: What decisions have they made for you?

The essence of the criterion is that one encourages or allows others to assume responsibility for most major areas of one's life, such as decisions about the selection of schools, occupation, place of employment, spouse, friends, place of residence, etc. Merely seeking advice or reassurance is not within the scope of the criterion. The subject must abdicate responsibility for the decisions and leave them for others to make. The criterion should be applied conservatively to those under 25 years of age. Allowance should also be made for obvious ethnic and cultural factors.

2   Has allowed others to make several important decisions in at least two different areas of life.

1   Has allowed others to make at least two major decisions in one or more areas of life.

0   Denied or examples unconvincing.

11.   0   1   2   ?   **0**   **1**   **2**
Difficulty in maintaining any course of action that offers no immediate reward
Emotionally unstable; Impulsive type: 4

Do you have trouble sticking with a plan or course of action, if you don't get something out of it right away?
If yes: Does that ever cause problems for you or get you into trouble?
  If yes: Give me some examples.

This refers to impatience and lack of perseverance when there is no immediate reward. To be scored positively there must be evidence from convincing examples that this results in subjective distress or problems in social or occupational functioning. Impatience associated with the pursuit of minor, everyday matters is not within the scope of the criterion.

2   Frequently has difficulty maintaining any course of action that offers no immediate reward. This sometimes causes subjective distress or problems in social or occupational functioning.

1   Occasionally has difficulty maintaining any course of action that offers no immediate reward. This sometimes causes subjective distress or problems in social or occupational functioning.

0   Denied, rare, or examples unconvincing.

12.   0   1   2   ?   **0   1   2**

Suggestibility (the individual is easily influenced by others or by circumstances)

Histrionic: 2

Are you easily influenced by other people's suggestions?
If yes: Do you ever go along with suggestions that get you into trouble?
  If yes: Give me some examples.

Are you easily influenced by what's going on around you?
If yes: Does that ever get you into trouble?
  If yes: Give me some examples.

The essence of the criterion is the ease and frequency with which one's behaviour is influenced by the conditions around one, or by the ideas and opinions of others rather than one's own. It is scored positively only if there are convincing examples that this suggestibility sometimes causes social or occupational problems.

2   Is frequently suggestible. This sometimes causes social or occupational problems.

1   Is occasionally suggestible. This sometimes causes social or occupational problems.

0   Denied, rare, or examples unconvincing.

13.　　0　1　2　?　　**0**　**1**　**2**
Belief that one is socially inept, personally unappealing, or inferior to others
Anxious [avoidant]:　2

Do you feel awkward or out of place in social situations?
If yes: Give me some examples of what you mean.

Do you believe that people find you uninteresting or unappealing?
If yes: Tell me about it.

Do you feel inferior to most people?
If yes: Why do you believe that?

Whether or not one is really socially inept, personally unappealing, or inferior to others is irrelevant. What counts is one's beliefs. All three aspects of the criterion are not required. It is particularly important to determine whether the beliefs are confined to isolated episodes of mental illness, in which case they are not scored as present.

2　Almost always feels socially inept, unappealing, or inferior to others

1　Often feels socially inept, unappealing, or inferior to others

0　Denied, rare, confined to isolated episodes of mental illness, or not supported by convincing examples

14.   0   1   2   ?   **0   1   2**
          Excessive conscientiousness and scrupulousness
          Anankastic: 4

Are morals and ethics much more important to you than they are to most people?
If yes: Including people from your own background or religion?
   If yes: Give me some examples of what you mean.

Are you (also) very concerned about rules and regulations?
If yes: Give me some examples.

Are you so strict or conscientious that you spend a lot of time worrying whether you have broken any rules or done something wrong?
If yes: Give me some examples.

If no: Have people accused you of being too strict or rigid about what's right and wrong?
   If yes: Why do you think they've said that?

It is not uncommon for people to view themselves as conscientious or subscribing to a higher morality than others. This is insufficient grounds for a positive rating. There must be evidence of an excessive concern about rules, ethics, morality, or matters of right and wrong. This may express itself in extreme rigidity and inflexibility about such matters, undue concern or preoccupation with doing what is right, or excessive worrying about having broken rules or done something immoral or unethical. It is not necessary that subjects impose their scrupulosity or rigidity on others. It is particularly important to view the subjects' behaviour within the context of their cultural background and religious beliefs or allegiances. Religious individuals should be judged in relation to others of the same sect, and scored positively only if members of the same religion would also view them as scrupulous or inflexible. The criterion should not be scored positively if the behaviour is present only during isolated episodes of depression or obsessive-compulsive disorder.

2   Usually is overconscientious, scrupulous, and inflexible about matters of morality, ethics, or values.

1   Occasionally is overconscientious, scrupulous, and inflexible about matters of morality, ethics, or values.

0   Denied, rare, confined to isolated episodes of depression or obsessive-compulsive disorder, or not supported by convincing examples.

*15.   0 1 2 ? **0** **1** **2**
     Very low tolerance to frustration
     Dissocial: 4 (partial)

Do you ever feel very frustrated or angry when you don't get what you want right away?
If yes: When that happens does it ever cause problems for you or get you into trouble?
 If yes: Give me some examples.

Subjects must indicate that they experience annoyance or anger when they cannot get what they want right away or have to wait too long for it. In order for the criterion to be scored positively the feeling of frustration must lead to behaviour that causes problems or gets the subject into trouble. The mere experience of anger or frustration is insufficient for a positive score.

2 Actions frequently directed toward obtaining immediate satisfaction, and feels frustrated when not immediately gratified. This sometimes leads to behaviour that causes social or occupational problems.

1 Actions occasionally directed toward obtaining immediate satisfaction, and feels frustrated when not immediately gratified. This sometimes leads to behaviour that causes social or occupational problems.

0 Denied, rare, does not cause social or occupational problems, or examples unconvincing.

---

16.   0   1   2   ?   **0   1   2**

Continual seeking for activities in which the individual is the centre of attention

Histrionic: 4 (partial)

Do you ever have a strong need to be the centre of attention?
If yes: Tell me about it.

How do you feel when you're not the centre of attention?

If no: Have people ever said you need to be the centre of attention?
  If yes: Why do you think they've said that?

It is normal to desire a certain amount of attention. The criterion refers only to those who have an almost insatiable need for it. This is manifest by the frequency with which they pursue behaviours that are intended to ensure that they are the centre of attention, and the discomfort of one form or another that they experience when too much time elapses without their receiving the attention they crave. The criterion is not scored 2 unless the subject acknowledges discomfort or distress, when the attention is not received.

Frequently has a very strong need to be the centre of attention. When the need is not gratified, there is sometimes an experience of considerable discomfort or distress.

1   Frequently has a very strong need to be the centre of attention. When the need is not gratified, there is rarely or never an experience of considerable discomfort or distress.

Occasionally has a very strong need to be the centre of attention. When the need is not gratified, there is sometimes an experience of considerable discomfort or distress.

0   Denied, the need for attention is reasonable, or the examples are unconvincing.

17.   0   1   2   ?   **0**   **1**   **2**

Over-concern with physical attractiveness

Histrionic: 6

How important to you is your physical appearance?

Do you like to dress so that you stand out in a crowd?

Do you ever try to use your physical appearance to attract attention?
If yes: Tell me more about it.

In rating this criterion also consider subject's appearance during interview.

The essence of the criterion is the use of one's physical appearance as a means of drawing attention to oneself. Denial of the behaviour and obvious manifestation of it in the interview may be used as the basis for a positive rating, including a score of 2 if it is very striking and not due to hypomania.

2   Frequently uses physical appearance to draw attention to self.

Denied but very striking in interview.

1   Occasionally uses physical appearance to draw attention to self.

Denied but somewhat present in interview

0   Rarely or never uses physical appearance to draw attention to self.

---

18.   0   1   2   ?   **0**   **1**   **2**
Excessive preoccupation with fantasy and introspection
Schizoid: 7

Do you get much more enjoyment from daydreaming than you do from real life?
If yes: Tell me about it.

Do you (also) prefer to be alone with your own thoughts, rather than involved with other people or with what's going on around you?
If yes: Tell me about it.

This concerns a detachment from the outer world in favor of one's own inner mental life. In order to be scored 2 subjects should make it very clear that they overwhelmingly prefer or enjoy being alone with their own thoughts and imagination, rather than involved with other people and with what is going on in the world around them.

2   Overwhelmingly prefers to spend time with own thoughts or imagination, rather than with other people and with what is going on in environment.

1   Prefers, but not overwhelmingly so, to spend time with own thoughts or imagination rather than with other people and with what is going on in environment.

0   Denied, acknowledged but not supported by subject's description, or fantasy life and introspective reserve are not prominent.

III. INTERPERSONAL RELATIONSHIPS

Now I would like to talk to you about the people in your life. Remember I'm interested in what has been typical of you throughout your life and not just recently, but if you have changed and are different from the way you used to be, be sure to let me know.

Who are the most important people in your life?

In what way are they important?

During your life what kind of problems or difficulties have you had getting along with other people?

---

19.   0   1   2   ?   **0   1   2**
No desire for, or possession of, any close friends or confiding relationships (or only one)
Schizoid: 8

Do you have any close friends or people you confide in?
If yes: Tell me about them.

If no: Would you like to?
  If yes: Tell me about it.
  If no: Is there anyone you have ever been close to or confided in?
    If yes: Tell me about it.

The criterion also requires no desire for close friendships or confiding relationships, and not merely their absence from one's life.

2   Neither desires nor has any close friends or confidants (or only one).

1   Probably neither desires nor has any close friends or confidants (or only one), but there is some doubt about this based on the subject's uncertainty or description of the nature of the friendships.

0   Denied or description unconvincing.

20.   0   1   2   ?   NA   **0   1   2**
Incapacity to maintain enduring relationships, though with no difficulty in establishing them
Dissocial: 3

If 19 was scored 2, circle NA and go to 21.

How long have these relationships lasted?

To be scored positively there should be convincing evidence from examples that the subject has an inability to sustain friendships and relationships with others, excluding family members. In this context a spouse is not considered a family member. Not scored positively are those who claim never to establish friendships or relationships in the first place (**NA**), and those who through misfortune or events beyond their control (deaths, illness, moving, etc.) report the interruption of many relationships. Five years is considered evidence of an enduring relationship.

2   The subject has never maintained an enduring or longstanding relationship with anyone (excluding family members) since the completion of childhood.

1   The subject has maintained an enduring or longstanding relationship with only one person (excluding family members) since the completion of childhood.

Examples suggest the likelihood that the subject has never maintained an enduring or longstanding relationship (excluding family members) since the completion of childhood, but they are less than totally convincing.

0   Denied, not supported by examples, or due to circumstances beyond the subject's control.

---

21.   0   1   2   ?   **0**   **1**   **2**

Avoidance of social activities that involve significant interpersonal contact, because of fear of criticism, disapproval, or rejection

Anxious [avoidant]:   6 (partial)

Some people almost always keep to themselves and rarely socialize. Are you like that?
If yes: Tell me more about it.

Why do you think you behave like that?

For a positive score there must be evidence of an obvious avoidance of joint leisure activities, social visits, parties, or participation in community, civic, or other organizations. Social contacts at work or with one's family do not exempt one from meeting the criterion. The reason for the avoidance must be fear of criticism, disapproval or rejection.

2   Almost always avoids social activities (outside of family or work) that involve significant interpersonal contact. Subject provides one or more of these as the primary reason: fear of criticism, disapproval or rejection.

1   Often avoids social activities (outside of family or work) that involve significant interpersonal contact. Subject provides one or more of these as the primary reason: fear of criticism, disapproval or rejection.

Almost always avoids social activities (outside of family or work) that involve significant interpersonal contact. Subject acknowledges one or more of the three reasons, but insists that they are not the primary reasons.

0   Denied, infrequent, not supported by convincing examples, or avoidance is due to other reasons.

22.   0   1   2   ?   **0**   **1**   **2**
              Consistent choice of solitary activities
              Schizoid: 6

Do you almost always choose the kind of activities that you can do all by yourself rather than with other people?
If yes: Give me some examples.

For a score of 2 there must be compelling evidence from examples that sub-jects almost always select activities (occupational and leisure) that they can do alone. The mere preference for such activities is insufficient. It must be acted on. Those who almost always choose solitary leisure activities but claim that their job occasionally prevents them from choosing solitary occupational activities should receive a score of 2.

2   Almost always chooses solitary occupational and leisure activities.

     Almost always chooses solitary occupational and leisure activities, except occa-sionally when the nature of the job prevents it.

1   Often chooses solitary occupational and leisure activities.

0   Denied or examples unconvincing.

23.   0   1   2   ?   **0   1   2**

Unwillingness to become involved with people unless certain of being liked

Anxious [avoidant]:   4

Are you willing to get involved with people when you're not sure they really like you?

If no: Does that affect you or the way you live your life?

   If yes: Tell me about it.

     Many people acknowledge this tendency, but that is insufficient for a positive score. For a score of 2 the subject's description must make it clear that it has a significant impact, e.g., missing out on opportunities for potential friendships and relationships.

2   Usually unwilling to become involved with people unless certain of being liked, and this has an obvious effect on friendships and relationships.

1   Occasionally unwilling to become involved with people unless certain of being liked, and this has some effect on friendships and relationships.

0   Denied, rare, or not supported by description.

24.   0   1   2   ?   **0**   **1**   **2**

Excessive preoccupation with being criticized or rejected in social situations

Anxious [avoidant]:   3

Do you spend a lot of time worrying about whether people like you?

If yes: Are you afraid they'll criticize or reject you when you're around them?

  If yes: How much does this bother you?

There is an inclination for subjects to confuse an ordinary, understandable concern about criticism or rejection in social situations with an excessive preoccupation. It is particularly important that acknowledgement of the behaviour be supported by convincing examples indicating that the concern is well beyond that experienced by most people in similar circumstances.

2   Frequently is concerned about being criticized or rejected in social situations.

1   Occasionally is concerned about being criticized or rejected in social situations.

0   Denied, rare, or not supported by convincing examples.

25.   0   1   2   ?   **0**   **1**   **2**
Disburtances in and uncertainty about internal preferences
Emotionally unstable; Borderline type: 1 (partial)

Do you have a lot of trouble deciding what type of friends you should have?
If yes: Does that have an effect on your life or cause any problems for you?
   If yes: Give me some examples.

Does the kind of people you have as friends keep changing?
If yes: Tell me about it.

This aspect of the criterion is met when subjects report that they are so uncertain about what type of friends they desire, that this causes significant distress or problems in their relations with others. A positive score is also given when subjects describes frequent or erratic changes in the type of friends they have, even if they don't acknowledge uncertainty about type of friends to have. Doubt about whether to have a particular person as a friend is not within the scope of the criterion, unless it is a particular instance of the more general uncertainty about the *type* of friends to have.

2   Obvious and well documented persistent uncertainty about type of friends to have, as described above.

1   Probable but less well documented persistent uncertainty about type of friends to have, as described above.

0   Absent, doubtful, or not well documented by examples.

*26.   0   1   2   ?   **0**   **1**   **2**
Liability to become involved in intense and unstable relationships often leading to emotional crises
Emotionally unstable; Borderline type: 2

Do you get into intense and stormy relationships with other people with lots of ups and downs? I mean where your feelings about them run "hot" and "cold," or change from one extreme to the other.
If yes: In those relationships do you often find yourself alternating between admiring and despising the same person?
  If yes: Give me some examples.

In how many different relationships has this happened?

For a positive score three features must be present: instability, strong feelings, and alternation between overidealization and devaluation. The latter does not require continuous switching from overidealization to devaluation. If the other requirements are met, it does not matter whether the behaviour is confined to specific types of relationships, e.g., those with parents, members of the opposite sex, etc.

2   Examples illustrating a pattern of unstable and intense relationships (more than one or two) characterized by alternating between the extremes of overidealization and devaluation.

1   Examples illustrating that one or two relationships were unstable, intense and characterized by alternating between the extremes of overidealization and devaluation.

0   Denied or not supported by convincing examples.

27.   0   1   2   ?   **0   1   2**
Unreasonable insistence by the individual that others submit to exactly his or her way of doing things, or unreasonable reluctance to allow others to do things
Anankastic:: 8

Do you often insist that people do things exactly your way?
If yes: Does that cause any problems for you or for others?
          If yes: Tell me about it.

Are you reluctant to let people do things, because you're convinced that they won't do them your way?
If yes: Does that cause any problems for you or for them?
  If yes: Tell me about it.

For a positive score the behaviour must cause subjective distress or problems.

2   Frequent insistence that others submit to exactly his or her way of doing things. This sometimes causes subjective distress or problems.

Frequent unreasonable reluctance to allow others to do things because of the conviction that they will not do them correctly. This sometimes causes subjective distress or problems.

1   Occasional insistence that others submit to exactly his or her way of doing things. This sometimes causes subjective distress or problems.

Occasional unreasonable reluctance to allow others to do things because of the conviction that they will not do them correctly. This sometimes causes subjective distress or problems.

0   Denied, does not cause distress or problems, or not supported by convincing examples.

28.   0   1   2   ?   **0**   **1**   **2**
Rigidity and stubbornness
Anankastic: 7

Are you very stubborn and set in your ways?
If yes: Give me some examples of what you mean.

Does this upset you or cause any problems?

If no: Have people ever accused you of being that way?
  If yes: Why do you think they have?

Resistance to the suggestions and views of others, and a reluctance to change one's ways under reasonable pressure from others to do so, should be taken as evidence of rigidity and stubbornness. For a positive score there should be indications that this sometimes leads to subjective distress or social or occupational problems.

2   Frequent rigidity and stubbornness that sometimes leads to subjective distress or social or occupational problems.

1   Occasional rigidity and stubbornness that sometimes leads to subjective distress or social or occupational problems.

0   Denied, not associated with subjective distress or social or occupational problems.

29.   0   1   2   ?   **0   1   2**
Callous unconcern for the feelings of others
Dissocial: 1

Some people are not too concerned about other people's feelings. Are you like that?
If yes: Tell me more about it.

If no: Has anyone ever told you that you're not concerned about other people's feelings?
   If yes: Why do you think they've said that?

Many callous people may be unaware of it or fail to acknowledge it. Therefore, it is particularly important to adequately pursue the reasons for any accusations by others.

2   Usually is not concerned about the feelings of others.
1   Often is not concerned about the feelings of others.
0   Denied, infrequent, or not supported by examples.

---

30.   0   1   2   ?   **0   1   2**
**Marked tendency to quarrelsome behaviour and to conflicts with oth-
ers, especially when impulsive acts are thwarted or criticized**
Emotionally unstable; Impulsive type: 2

Do you have a habit of getting into arguments and disagreements?
If yes: When are you likely to behave like that?

Give me some examples.

If no: Have people told you that you argue or disagree too much?
          If yes: Why do you think they have?

To receive a positive score there must be evidence from examples that the
quarrelsome behaviour and conflicts occur especially when the subject's
impulsive acts are prevented, condemned, or criticized.

2   Frequently engages in quarrelsome behaviour and conflicts with others, espe-
     cially when impulsive acts are prevented, condemned, or criticized.

1   Occasionally engages in quarrelsome behaviour and conflicts with others,
     especially when impulsive acts are prevented, condemned, or criticized.

     Frequently engages in quarrelsome behaviour and conflicts with others, but
     not especially in relation to impulsive acts.

0   Denied, rare, not in relation to impulsive acts, or not supported by convincing
     examples.

31.   0   1   2   ?   **0**   **1**   **2**
A combative and tenacious sense of personal rights out of keeping with the actual situation
Paranoid: 4

Do you insist on standing up for your rights?
If yes: Do you do this even when it means getting into a confrontation and arguing about something that many people would ignore?
  If yes: Give me some examples.

If no: Have people accused you of being like that?
  If yes: Why do you think they have?

Argumentative or disagreeable behaviour is not within the scope of the criterion, unless it occurs within the context of subjects' defending in an exaggerated or inappropriate fashion what they perceive to be their rights.

2   Frequently displays a combative and tenacious sense of personal rights out of keeping with the actual situation.

1   Occasionally displays a combative and tenacious sense of personal rights out of keeping with the actual situation.

0   Denied, rare, or not supported by convincing examples.

32.   0   1   2   ?   NA   **0   1   2**
Unwillingness to make even reasonable demands on the people one depends on
Dependent: 3

Do you depend a lot on some people?
If no: Score 32 and 33 NA, and go to 34.
If yes: Do you ask them to help you or do things for you?
   Tell me about it.

This refers specifically to reasonable demands on the people the subject depends on, e.g., spouse, parents, adult offspring, lover, friends, etc. It does not include such behaviour when it occurs with an employer, or outside the context of dependent relationships.

2   Usually unwilling to make even reasonable demands on the people the subject depends on.

1   Occasionally unwilling to make even reasonable demands on the people the subject depends on.

0   Denied, rare, or not supported by convincing examples.

33.	0	1	2	?	NA	**0**	**1**	**2**

Subordination of one's own needs to those of others on whom one is dependent, and undue compliance with their wishes

Dependent: 2

When you depend a lot on another person, do you give in too easily to what that person wants?
If yes: Give me some examples of what you mean.

Do you almost always put that person's needs ahead of your own?
If yes: Tell me about it.

As with the preceding item (**32**) this applies only to behaviour that occurs with those on whom the subject is dependent, e.g., spouse, parents, adult off-spring, lover, friends, etc. It does not include such behaviour when it occurs with an employer, or outside the context of dependent relationships.

2 Frequently subordinates own needs to those on whom subject is dependent, or unduly complies with their wishes.

1 Occasionally subordinates own needs to those on whom subject is dependent, or unduly complies with their wishes.

0 Denied, rare, or not supported by convincing examples.

*34.   0   1   2   ?   **0   1   2**

Tendency to bear grudges persistently, e.g., refusal to forgive insults injuries, or slights

Paranoid: 2

Have you ever held a grudge or taken a long time to forgive someone?
If yes: Tell me about it.

Did you try to avoid or refuse to talk to the person?

How long did you continue to act that way?

Has this ever happened with anyone else?
If yes: With how many people?

As evidence of a grudge the subject should either try to avoid or refuse to speak to the person for more than a year. For a score of 2 there should be evidence of grudges against more than one or two people. The examples should establish that the reaction is obviously disproportionate. For example, a grudge against a parent responsible for child abuse or incest would not warrant a positive score.

2   Has born persistent grudges, i.e., has been unforgiving of insults, injuries, or slights against several people.

1   Has born persistent grudges, i.e., has been unforgiving of insults, injuries, or slights against one or two people.

0   Denied or not supported by example

---

35.   0   1   2   ?   **0   1   2**
Suspiciousness and a pervasive tendency to distort experience by misconstruing the neutral or friendly actions of others as hostile or contemptuous
Paranoid: 3

Has it been your experience that people often try to use you or take advantage of you?
If yes: Give me some examples.

Has anyone ever deliberately tried to harm you, ruin your reputation, or make life difficult for you?
If yes: Give me some examples.

In rating this criterion also consider subject's behaviour during interview.

Affirmative replies to the questions that assess this criterion require considerable probing and judgment on the part of the examiner, because there must be an assessment of the possible reality basis of the subject's reported experiences. Too much emphasis should not be given to accounts of isolated incidents. The focus should be on identifying a characteristic attitude on the part of the subject, suggesting an orientation or set toward the expectation of exploitation or harm. The subject's approach to the interview itself may be taken into consideration in the scoring, but should never be the sole basis for a score of 2.

2   Frequently expects, without sufficient basis, to be exploited or harmed by others.

1   Occasionally expects, without sufficient basis, to be exploited or harmed by others.

Denied, but evident in interview.

0   Denied, rare, or not supported by convincing examples.

36.   0   1   2   ?   **0**   **1**   **2**
Persistent self-referential attitude, associated particularly with excessive self-importance
Paranoid: 6

When you enter a room full of people do you often wonder whether they might be talking about you, or even making unflattering remarks about you?
If yes: Give me some examples.

When you're in a public place or walking down the street, do you often wonder whether people might be looking at you, talking about you, or even making fun of you?
If yes: Give me some examples.

It is not uncommon for people to experience fleeting self-referential ideas when they first enter a large social gathering, particularly one involving unfamiliar people. Such behaviour should not be considered within the scope of the criterion. There should be indications that the ideas are more than momentary. If it appears that they may be of delusional proportions, the subject should be questioned carefully, since delusions of reference are excluded.

2   Frequently experiences ideas of reference.

1   Occasionally experiences ideas of reference.

0   Denied, rare, not supported by convincing examples, or delusional in nature.

IV. AFFECTS

Now I am going to ask some questions about your feelings. Again I'm interested in the way you have been most of your life and not just recently. If you have changed and are different from the way you used to be, be sure to let me know.

How do you usually feel?

How do you usually feel deep down inside?

What problems do you have with your feelings?

---

37.   0   1   2   ?   **0   1   2**
            An appearance of indifference to either praise or criticism
            Schizoid: 4

When you're praised, do you show any reaction so that the people around you know how you feel?
If yes: Tell me about it.

What about when you're criticized?
If yes: Tell me about it.

For a positive score subjects must report the absence of any overt reaction, so that observers might conclude that they are indifferent to the praise or criticism. Apparent indifference to both praise and criticism is not required.

2   Almost always gives the appearance of being indifferent to praise or criticism.

1   Often gives the appearance of being indifferent to praise or criticism.

0   Denied, does not occur often, or not supported by subject's account.

38.   0   1   2   ?   **0   1   2**
Excessive sensitivity to setbacks and rebuffs
Paranoid: 1

Are you easily slighted or offended?
If yes: Tell me about it.

When you are slighted or offended, do you sometimes have too strong a reaction?
If yes: Give me some examples.

How do you react when things don't go your way?

For a positive score the subject's examples should establish the presence of a characteristic inclination toward being slighted in situations where most people would not especially feel that way; or of reacting excessively to actual slights. This may occur as a consequence of what others say or fail to say, or what they do or fail to do. For a 2 score there must also be evidence of similar behaviour in response to setbacks, i.e., things not going one's way.

2   Frequently is easily slighted, or reacts excessively to actual slights. Also displays similar behaviour in response to setbacks.

1   Occasionally is easily slighted, or reacts excessively to actual slights. Also displays similar behaviour in response to setbacks.

Frequently is easily slighted, or reacts excessively to actual slights, but not to setbacks.

Frequently reacts excessively to setbacks, but not slights.

0   Denied, rare, or not supported by convincing examples.

39.	0	1	2	?	**0**	**1**	**2**

Limited capacity to express warm, tender feelings towards others
Schizoid: 3 (partial)

Some people rarely show affection or talk about it. Are you like that?
If yes: Tell me about it.

If no: Have people told you that you're not affectionate?
   If yes: Why do you think they've said that?

Warmth, tenderness, or affection are the only emotions within the scope of the criterion, which concerns their display or expression, not the subjective experience of them.

2   Claims to rarely or never express affection.

1   Claims to occasionally express affection.

0   Frequently expresses affection.

---

40.   0   1   2   ?   **0**   **1**   **2**
         Self-dramatization, theatricality, or exaggerated expression of emotions
         Histrionic: 1

Do you almost always show your feelings in a very obvious way for others to see?
If yes: Do you ever get carried away and exaggerate the way you feel?
   If yes: Give me some examples.

Have people told you that you're dramatic?
If yes: Why do you think they've said that?

In rating this criterion also consider subject's behaviour during interview.

 Subjects should be questioned very closely if they acknowledge self-dramatization, but show no signs of it during the interview. Strikingly obvious theatricality or frequent exaggerated expression of emotions during the interview may justify a positive rating, including a score of 2, even if the subject denies the behaviour, provided there is no reason to suspect hypomania.

2   Acknowledges with supporting examples frequent self-dramatization and exaggerated expression of emotion, or displays it during the interview in an obvious and striking way.

1   Acknowledges with supporting examples occasional self-dramatization and exaggerated expression of emotion, or displays it to a limited degree during the interview.

0   Denied, rare, or not supported by convincing examples or behaviour during the interview.

---

41.   0   1   2   ?   **0**   **1**   **2**
Continual seeking for excitement
Histrionic: 4 (partial)

Do you need a lot of excitement in your life?
If yes: Tell me more about it.

Does needing excitement ever cause problems for you?
If yes: Give me some examples.

Proneness to boredom without obvious seeking of excitement is not within the scope of the criterion. For a positive score there should be evidence that the search for exciting forms of behaviour sometimes causes problems for the subject.

2   Frequently seeks excitement. This leads to the pursuit of exciting forms of behaviour that sometimes cause problems for the subject.

1   Occasionally seeks excitement. This leads to the pursuit of exciting forms of behaviour that sometimes cause problems for the subject.

0   Denied, not supported by subject's description, or rarely or never leads to exciting forms of behaviour that cause problems for the subject.

---

42.   0   1   2   ?   **0   1   2**
Few, if any, activities provide pleasure
Schizoid: 1

Are there any activities that you enjoy?
If yes: Tell me about them.

If no: Tell me more about it.

It is particularly important to establish that the anhedonia is not limited to episodes of depression. Positive ratings should also not be given to those with dysthymia or persistent depression.

2   Claims to rarely, if ever, experience pleasure or joy.

1   Claims not to experience pleasure or joy most of the time.

0   Denied, infrequent, due to depression, or not supported by subject's description.

43.   0   1   2   ?   **0**   **1**   **2**
Liability to outbursts of anger or violence, with inability to control the resulting behavioural explosions
Emotionally unstable; Impulsive type: 3

Do you sometimes get angrier than you should, or feel very angry without a good reason?
If yes: Give me some examples.

If no: Have people ever told you that you're a very angry person?
   If yes: Why do you think they've said that?

Do you ever lose your temper and have tantrums or angry outbursts?
If yes: Do you yell and scream in an uncontrolled way?
   If yes: Give me some examples.

Do you ever throw, break, or smash things?
If yes: Give me some examples.

Do you ever hit or assault people?
If yes: Give me some examples.

The subjective experience of intense anger or psychodynamically inferred anger are not within the scope of the criterion. The anger must be either inappropriate, or intense and uncontrolled. Overt verbal or physical displays of anger are required.

2   Frequently verbally displays inappropriate or intense, uncontrolled anger.

Occasionally indulges in extreme physical displays of inappropriate or intense, uncontrolled anger.

1   Occasionally verbally displays inappropriate or intense, uncontrolled anger.

On one or two occasions indulged in extreme physical displays of inappropriate or intense, uncontrolled anger.

0   Denied.

44. 0 1 2 ?   **0** **1** **2**
Limited capacity to express anger towards others
Schizoid: 3 (partial)

If 43 is scored 1 or 2, score 44 0 and go to 45.

When you're angry with someone, do you show it so that the person is aware of it?
Tell me more about it

This concerns the expression or display and not the experience of anger toward others.

2 Claims to almost never express anger toward others, so that they are aware of it.

1 Claims to rarely express anger toward others, so that they are aware of it.

0 Expresses anger toward others or claim not supported by subject's account.

45.   0   1   2   ?   **0**   **1**   **2**

Chronic feelings of emptiness
Emotionally unstable; Borderline type: 5

Do you often feel empty inside?
If yes: Does that upset you or cause any problems for you?
  If yes: Tell me about it.

For a positive score there must be evidence that the emptiness is obviously distressing to the subject or leads to maladaptive behaviour, e.g., substance abuse, self-mutilation, suicidal gestures, impulsive sexual activity, etc.

2   Frequent feelings of emptiness that are obviously distressing or sometimes lead to maladaptive behaviour.

1   Occasional feelings of emptiness that are obviously distressing or sometimes lead to maladaptive behaviour.

0   Denied, rare, or not associated with obvious distress or maladaptive behaviour.

46. 　　0　1　2　?　　**0　1　2**

Feeling uncomfortable or helpless when alone, because of exaggerated fears of inability to care for oneself
Dependent:　4

How do you usually feel when you're alone?

If subject reports uncomfortable or helpless feelings:
How much of a problem is that? How much does it actually bother you?

Why do you think you feel that way?

　　　　For a positive score subjects must experience significant and obvious discomfort or helplessness when alone, or provide convincing examples that they go to great lengths to avoid being alone. The reason for this must be a fear of being unable to care for oneself. A feeling of loneliness as such does not receive a positive score.

2　Frequently feels very uncomfortable or helpless when alone, because of exaggerated fear of inability to care for oneself.

1　Occasionally feels very uncomfortable or helpless when alone, because of exaggerated fear of inability to care for oneself.

0　Denied, rare, feelings insignificant, not supported by subject's description, or solely for other reasons, e.g., loneliness.

47.   0   1   2   ?   **0   1   2**
            Preoccupation with fears of being left to care for oneself
            Dependent: 5

Do you spend a lot of time worrying about the possibility that you may be left alone and have to care for yourself?
If yes: Tell me about it.

The criterion refers to a fear and not the actual event. An occasional or transient concern is not within the scope of the criterion. There must be a long-standing preoccupation, not limited to an episode of illness. Positive scores should not be given if the preoccupation is due to special circumstances, such as those created by the serious illness or impending death of another, or the absence of other support systems, such as might occur in an elderly person with no surviving friends or family members.

2   Frequent unrealistic preoccupation with fears of being left to care for oneself.

1   Occasional unrealistic preoccupation with fears of being left to care for oneself.

0   Denied, rare, not supported by subject's description, or the fears have a definite basis in reality.

---

48.   0   1   2   ?   **0**   **1**   **2**
Excessive efforts to avoid abandonment
Emotionally unstable; Borderline type: 3

Do you ever find yourself frantically trying to stop someone close to you from leaving you?
If yes: Give me some examples.

Unlike the previous Dependent item (**47**), which concerns preoccupation with fears of being left alone to care for oneself, this has to do with efforts on the part of the subject to avoid real or imagined abandonment. The efforts should be associated with obvious feelings of anxiety or agitation.

2   Frequent frantic efforts to avoid real or imagined abandonment.

1   Occasional frantic efforts to avoid real or imagined abandonment.

0   Denied, rare, occurs only in association with suicidal or self-mutilating behaviour, or not supported by examples.

---

49.   0   1   2   ?   **0**   **1**   **2**
               Shallow and labile affectivity
               Histrionic: 3

Do your feelings often change very suddenly and unexpectedly, sometimes for no obvious reason?
If yes: Give me some examples.

Has anyone ever accused you of being a shallow person?
If yes: Why do you think they have?

In rating this criterion also consider subject's behaviour during interview.

Unlike the next item (**50**), the emotions involved are not necessarily negative ones, such as anxiety, depression, and irritability, but may include enthusiasm, warmth, joy, etc. Denial of the behaviour and display of it in the interview is insufficient for a score of 2. Do not give a positive rating when the behaviour is due to a bipolar disorder.

2   Frequently displays rapidly shifting and shallow expression of emotions.

1   Occasionally displays rapidly shifting and shallow expression of emotions.

     Denied, but definitely displayed during interview.

0   Denied, rare, not supported by convincing examples, or due to a bipolar disorder.

50.   0   1   2   ?   **0**   **1**   **2**
               Unstable and capricious mood
               Emotionally unstable; Impulsive type: 5

Do you often change from your usual mood to feeling very irritable, very depressed, or very nervous?
If yes: When that happens how long do you usually stay that way?

Give me some examples of what it's like when you're feeling that way.

The subject need not report instability of all three moods: depression, irritability, and anxiety. For a positive score the description and examples should establish that the mood changes are not only frequent and shortlived (a few hours or days), but also of some intensity.

2   Frequently experiences affective instability.

1   Occasionally experiences affective instability.

0   Denied, rare, or not supported by examples.

51.   0   1   2   ?   **0   1   2**
Restrictions in lifestyle because of need for physical security
Anxious [avoidant]:   5

Some people have a very strong need to feel safe from physical harm. That may affect the way they live their lives or prevent them from doing a lot of things. Are you like that?
If yes: Give me some examples.

The restrictions on the way subjects live their life because of the need for physical security may involve a variety of areas: social, leisure, and occupational. A positive score requires documentation with obvious examples. Vague generalities are insufficient.

2   The need for physical security has an obvious effect on the subject's lifestyle as reflected by convincing examples from different areas of life.

1   The need for physical security has a definite but less extensive effect on the subject's lifestyle.

0   Denied, insignificant, or not supported by convincing examples.

52.   0   1   2   ?   **0   1   2**
Persistent and pervasive feelings of tension and apprehension
Anxious [avoidant]:   1

Do you almost always feel tense or nervous?
If yes: How much of an effect does it have on your life?

Give me some examples.

Are you the kind of person who is always worrying that something bad or unpleasant is going to happen?
If yes: Is it very hard for you to get those thoughts out of your mind?
    If yes: How much of an effect does being a worrier have on your life?

A positive rating should not be given if the tension and apprehension are limited to isolated episodes of depressive, anxiety, phobic, panic, or obsessive-compulsive disorders. However, those with chronic anxiety disorders fall within the scope of the criterion. There must be convincing evidence that both tension and apprehension have an obvious effect on the subject's life.

2   Frequent experience of persistent and pervasive feelings of both tension and apprehension with an obvious effect on the subject's life.

1   Frequent experience of persistent and pervasive feelings of either tension or apprehension (but not both), with an obvious effect on the subject's life.

Occasional experience of persistent and pervasive feelings of both tension and apprehension with an obvious effect on the subject's life.

0   Denied, rare, confined to episodic anxiety or depressive disorders, does not have an obvious effect on the subject's life, or not supported by subject's description.

53. 0   1   2   ?   **0   1   2**
**Little interest in having sexual experiences with another person
(taking into account age)**
Schizoid: 5

The examiner should exercise discretion about inquiring about sexual behaviour in certain cultures. Where this might be inappropriate, the item should be scored ?

Now a few questions about your sexual behaviour. There are some people who have little or no desire to have sexual experiences with another person. Are you like that?
If yes: Tell me about it.

The lack of sexual interest or desire should be longstanding and not due to old age or to physical or mental illness, including depression. Allowance should also be made for the possible effect of certain medications.

2   Almost never has any desire to have sexual experiences with another person.

1   Much of the time has no desire to have sexual experiences with another person.

0   Denied, does not occur much of the time, explicable by age, physical or mental illness, medications, or not supported by subject's description.

---

54.   0   1   2   ?   **0   1   2**
Inappropriate seductiveness in appearance or behaviour
Histrionic: 5

---

he examiner should exercise discretion about inquiring about sexual behaviour in
certain cultures. Where this might be inappropriate, the item should be scored ?.

Do you ever find yourself dressing or behaving in a sexually seductive way?
If yes: What kind of things do you do?

Have you ever been told that what you do is inappropriate?
If yes: Tell me about it.

If no: Have you ever been told that you do?
  If yes: Why do you think people have said that?

In rating criterion also consider subject's appearance or behaviour during interview.

For a score of 2 the subject must provide examples of obviously inappropriate
seductiveness. The subject's appearance or behaviour during the interview
may influence the rating, and may be sufficient for a score of 2, if it is not due
to hypomania.

2   Frequently inappropriately sexually seductive in appearance or behaviour.

Obviously inappropriately seductive in appearance or behaviour during the
interview.

1   Occasionally inappropriately sexually seductive in appearance or behaviour.

Frequently either somewhat flirtatious or seductive in appearance or behaviour, but rarely inappropriately so.

Somewhat inappropriately seductive in appearance or behaviour during the
interview.

0   Denied, insignificant, or not supported by subject's description.

*55.　　0　1　2　?　　**0　1　2**
Recurrent suspicions, without justification, regarding sexual fidelity of spouse or sexual partner
Paranoid: 5

The examiner should exercise discretion about inquiring about sexual behaviour in certain cultures. Where this might be inappropriate, the item should be scored ?

Asked only of those who have never been married.
Have you ever had sexual relations with anyone?
If no: Circle NA and go to 56.

Have you ever been concerned about whether a sexual partner was unfaithful to you?
If yes: Tell me about it.

For a score of 2 there should be admission of more than brief, transient concerns about the sexual fidelity of one's spouse or partner. Subjects who admit to frequent suspicions, but who insist that it is justified, should be questioned very carefully. When in doubt about the possible reality basis of their account, the criterion should not be scored positively, unless there is evidence from other sources that the suspicions are pathological.

2　On a number of different occasions or with a number of different partners was obviously very concerned about fidelity, with no apparent justification.

1　On one or two occasions was obviously very concerned about fidelity, with no apparent justification.

0　Denied, rare, insignificant, or not supported by subject's account.

56.   0   1   2   ?   **0   1   2**
**Disturbances in and uncertainty about internal preferences
(including sexual)**
Emotionally unstable; Borderline type: 1 (partial)

**The examiner should exercise discretion about inquiring about sexual behaviour in
certain cultures. Where this might be inappropriate, the item should be scored ?**

Have you ever been uncertain whether you prefer a sexual relationship with a man or a
woman?
If yes: Tell me about it.

Does this ever upset you or cause any problems for you?
If yes: Tell me about it.

Homosexuality or bisexuality as such are not within the scope of the criterion
unless they are associated with significant doubt or uncertainty about one's
sexual orientation. This doubt or uncertainty causes subjective distress or
problems with others.

2   Has considerable doubt or uncertainty about sexual orientation. This frequently causes subjective distress.

1   Has considerable doubt or uncertainty about sexual orientation. This sometimes causes subjective distress.

0   Denied, rare, does not cause subjective distress, or not supported by subject's
account.

V. REALITY TESTING

Now a question about some of your beliefs.

---

57.   0   1   2   ?   **0   1   2**
Preoccupation with unsubstantiated "conspiratorial" explanations of events either immediate to the patient or in the world at large
Paranoid: 7

Do you spend time thinking about the possibility that there may be some kind of conspiracy going on around you or in the world at large?
If yes: Does this bother you or have any effect on your life?
   If yes: Tell me about it.

This should be scored conservatively. Passing suspicions or abstract ideas with little or no impact on the subject's behaviour are not within the scope of the criterion. For a positive score there should be a definite preoccupation that either produces emotional distress or has an obvious influence on the subject's behaviour. If people rather than events are the focus of the "conspiracy", then more than one person must be involved, and there must be communication between or among them.

2   Often preoccupied with unsubstantiated conspiratorial explanations. This sometimes produces emotional distress or has an obvious influence on the subject's behaviour.

1 Occasionally preoccupied with unsubstantiated conspiratorial explanations. This sometimes produces emotional distress or has an obvious influence on the subject's behaviour.

0   Denied, rare, does not cause distress or influence behaviour, or not supported by subject's description.

VI. IMPULSE CONTROL

I'm going to conclude the interview with some questions about impulsive and irresponsible behaviour. Have there been times when your behaviour hasn't conformed to what you believe or have been taught is right?
If yes: Tell me about it.

---

58.   0   1   2   ?   **0   1   2**
Marked tendency to act unexpectedly and without consideration of the consequences
Emotionally unstable; Impulsive type: 1

Some people have a habit of doing things suddenly or unexpectedly without giving any thought to what might happen. Are you like that?
If yes: What kind of things have you done?

This refers to the consequences of acting suddenly and unexpectedly on impulse. It is scored positively only if the subject can produce convincing examples of problems that have arisen or could have arisen as a result of this tendency.

2   Frequently acts suddenly and unexpectedly on impulse. This sometimes causes problems or could cause problems.

1   Occasionally acts suddenly and unexpectedly on impulse. This sometimes causes problems or could cause problems.

0   Denied, rare, or not supported by convincing examples.

*59.   0   1   2   ?   **0**   **1**   **2**
Recurrent threats or acts of self-harm
Emotionally unstable; Borderline type: 4

Have you ever threatened to commit suicide?
If yes: How many times?
   Tell me about it.

Have you ever actually made a suicide attempt or gesture?
If yes: How many times?
   Tell me about it.

Have you ever deliberately cut yourself, smashed your fist through a window, burned yourself, or hurt yourself in some other way (not counting suicide attempts or gestures)?
If yes: Tell me about it.

The mere sharing of one's suicidal thoughts with another person does not ordinarily constitute a threat. There must be communication of an intent to commit suicide. The motive for making the threat is irrelevant. Suicidal gestures are counted whether or not they were serious or accompanied by a genuine wish to die. Acts of self-harm include wrist cutting, deliberately breaking glass with one's body, burning oneself, headbanging, and other deliberate forms of self-injury of a nonsuicidal nature.

2   On several occasions engaged in suicidal threats, gestures, or acts of self-harm.

1   Once or twice engaged in suicidal threats, gestures, or acts of self-harm.

0   Denied.

*60.   0   1   2   ?   **0   1   2**
A low threshold for discharge of aggression, including violence
Dissocial: 4 (partial)

Have you ever hit or physically abused anyone in your family?
If yes: How many times?
  Tell me about it

Have you ever hit anyone (else) or been in any (other) fights?
If yes: How many times?
  Tell me about it.

Do not count aggression or violence associated with legitimate efforts at defending oneself or others. Alcohol and drugs are not exonerating factors.

2   Several times has been involved in physical fights, assaults, or physical abuse of others.

1   Once or twice has been involved in physical fights, assaults, or physical abuse of others.

0   Denied, or required by job or to defend someone or oneself.

*61.   0   1   2   ?   NA   **0   1   2**
Gross and persistent attitude of irresponsibility and disregard for social norms, rules, and obligations
Dissocial: 2

Have you ever been unemployed?
If yes: For how long?
   Why?

Have you ever traveled from place to place without a job or definite purpose or clear idea of when the travel would end?
If yes: Tell me about it.

Have you ever defaulted on debts or failed to honor financial obligations?
If yes: Tell me about it.

Have you ever failed to provide financial support for other members of your family, when you were expected to do so?
If yes: Tell me about it.

Asked only of those with children.
Have you ever failed to take adequate care of your children, or neglected their safety or physical well-being?
If yes: Tell me about it.

If no: Has anyone ever accused you of any of those things?
   If yes: Why do you think they have?

Asked only of males who have been separated or divorced.
Have you ever failed to provide alimony (financial maintenance) or child support payments when you were expected to?
If yes: Tell me about it.

Are you inclined to lie if it serves your purpose?
If yes: Give me some examples.

If no: Have people accused you of lying or not telling the truth?
   If yes: Why do you think they have?

Have you ever used an alias?
If yes: Why?

Have you ever "conned" anyone?
If yes: Tell me about it.

Do you ever take unnecessary chances and risk harm or injury to yourself or others?
If yes: Tell me about it.

Have you ever driven a car while you were intoxicated with alcohol or drugs?
If yes: How many times?
   Tell me about it.

Have you ever been stopped by the police for speeding or reckless driving (when you were not intoxicated with alcohol or drugs)?
If yes: How many times?
   Tell me about it.

Have you ever been arrested?
If yes: For what?

Have you ever done anything (else) that you could have been arrested for, if you had been caught?
If yes: What?

This criterion is rated based on the application of clinical judgment to the replies to the questions.

2   Convincing evidence of gross and persistent behaviour indicative of irresponsibility and disregard for social norms, rules, and obligations.

1   Suggestive but less than convincing evidence of gross and persistent behaviour indicative of irresponsibility and disregard for social norms, rules, and obligations.

0   No evidence or insufficient evidence for a positive rating.

---

62. 0   1   2   ?   NA   **0   1   2**
Incapacity to experience guilt
Dissocial: 5 (partial)

If 60 and 61 are both scored 0, score 62-64 NA, and go to 65.

How do you feel about **(cite behaviour acknowledged in items 60 and 61)**?

Do you think you were justified in behaving that way?

This criterion is rated based on a consideration of the history of dissocial behaviour viewed in conjunction with replies to questions regarding remorse or guilt. The examiner should cross-examine the subject closely to verify the authenticity of any alleged remorse or guilt. Regret because of the consequences for oneself, e.g., imprisonment, is not remorse. The rating should ultimately be based on the application of clinical judgment to all of this information.

2   Convincing evidence that the subject lacks remorse or the capacity to experience guilt.

1   Probable but less than convincing evidence that the subject lacks remorse or the capacity to experience guilt.

0   Appears to experience appropriate remorse or demonstrates the capacity to experience guilt.

63.   0   1   2   ?   NA   **0   1   2**

Marked proneness to blame others, or to offer plausible rationalizations for the behaviour that has brought the individual into conflict with society
          Dissocial: 6

Why do you think you behaved that way?

Be sure to confront subject with all areas and examples of dissocial behaviour.

The criterion is rated based on a consideration of the history of dissocial behaviour viewed in conjunction with the explanations of the behaviour offered by the subject. The examiner should cross-examine and confront the subject when necessary, to determine the validity of any attempts to blame others, or the plausibility of explanations for the behaviour. The rating is ultimately based on the application of clinical judgment to all of this information.

2   Convincing evidence that the subject is prone to blame others or to offer rationalizations for the dissocial behaviour.

1   Probable but less than convincing evidence that the subject is prone to blame others or to offer rationalizations for the dissocial behaviour.

0   Appears not to blame others or to offer rationalizations for the dissocial behaviour.

64.   0   1   2   ?   NA   **0   1   2**

Incapacity to profit from adverse experience, particularly punishment
Dissocial: 5 (partial)

The criterion is rated based on the application of clinical judgment to all of the information obtained in the interview that is relevant to the subject's history of dissocial behaviour.

2   Convincing evidence that the subject is unable to profit from experience, particularly punishment.

1   Probable but less than convincing evidence that the subject is unable to profit from experience, particularly punishment.

0   Appears to profit from experience, particularly punishment.

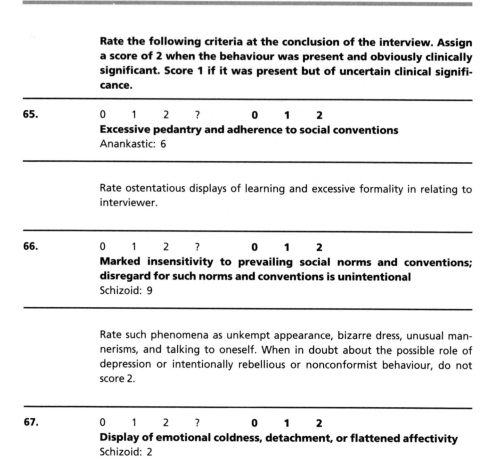

Rate the following criteria at the conclusion of the interview. Assign a score of 2 when the behaviour was present and obviously clinically significant. Score 1 if it was present but of uncertain clinical significance.

65.   0   1   2   ?   **0   1   2**
Excessive pedantry and adherence to social conventions
Anankastic: 6

Rate ostentatious displays of learning and excessive formality in relating to interviewer.

66.   0   1   2   ?   **0   1   2**
Marked insensitivity to prevailing social norms and conventions; disregard for such norms and conventions is unintentional
Schizoid: 9

Rate such phenomena as unkempt appearance, bizarre dress, unusual mannerisms, and talking to oneself. When in doubt about the possible role of depression or intentionally rebellious or nonconformist behaviour, do not score 2.

67.   0   1   2   ?   **0   1   2**
Display of emotional coldness, detachment, or flattened affectivity
Schizoid: 2

Rate unchanging facial expression, monotonous or unvarying vocal inflection, lack of expressive gestures, maintenance of a rigid, unchanging posture, poor eye contact, lack of apparent interest in examiner, failure to smile when almost everyone would. When in doubt about the presence or significance of these phenomena, including the possible role of psychotropic medications or depression, do not score 2.

IPDE ICD-10 module answer sheet

Last Name	First Name	Middle I.	Date

	Subject	Informant		Subject	Informant
1.	0 1 2 ? NA	0 1 2	**35.**	0 1 2 ?	0 1 2
2.	0 1 2 ?	0 1 2	**36.**	0 1 2 ?	0 1 2
3.	0 1 2 ?	0 1 2	**37.**	0 1 2 ?	0 1 2
4.	0 1 2 ?	0 1 2	**38.**	0 1 2 ?	0 1 2
5.	0 1 2 ?	0 1 2	**39.**	0 1 2 ?	0 1 2
6.	0 1 2 ?	0 1 2	**40.**	0 1 2 ?	0 1 2
7.	0 1 2 ?	0 1 2	**41.**	0 1 2 ?	0 1 2
8.	0 1 2 ?	0 1 2	**42.**	0 1 2 ?	0 1 2
9.	0 1 2 ?	0 1 2	**43.**	0 1 2 ?	0 1 2
10.	0 1 2 ?	0 1 2	**44.**	0 1 2 ?	0 1 2
11.	0 1 2 ?	0 1 2	**45.**	0 1 2 ?	0 1 2
12.	0 1 2 ?	0 1 2	**46.**	0 1 2 ?	0 1 2
13.	0 1 2 ?	0 1 2	**47.**	0 1 2 ?	0 1 2
14.	0 1 2 ?	0 1 2	**48.**	0 1 2 ?	0 1 2
15.	0 1 2 ?	0 1 2	**49.**	0 1 2 ?	0 1 2
16.	0 1 2 ?	0 1 2	**50.**	0 1 2 ?	0 1 2
17.	0 1 2 ?	0 1 2	**51.**	0 1 2 ?	0 1 2
18.	0 1 2 ?	0 1 2	**52.**	0 1 2 ?	0 1 2
19.	0 1 2 ?	0 1 2	**53.**	0 1 2 ?	0 1 2
20.	0 1 2 ?	0 1 2	**54.**	0 1 2 ?	0 1 2
21.	0 1 2 ? NA	0 1 2	**55.**	0 1 2 ? NA	0 1 2
22.	0 1 2 ?	0 1 2	**56.**	0 1 2 ?	0 1 2
23.	0 1 2 ?	0 1 2	**57.**	0 1 2 ?	0 1 2
24.	0 1 2 ?	0 1 2	**58.**	0 1 2 ?	0 1 2
25.	0 1 2 ?	0 1 2	**59.**	0 1 2 ?	0 1 2
26.	0 1 2 ?	0 1 2	**60.**	0 1 2 ?	0 1 2
27.	0 1 2 ?	0 1 2	**61.**	0 1 2 ? NA	0 1 2
28.	0 1 2 ?	0 1 2	**62.**	0 1 2 ? NA	0 1 2
29.	0 1 2 ?	0 1 2	**63.**	0 1 2 ? NA	0 1 2
30.	0 1 2 ?	0 1 2	**64.**	0 1 2 ? NA	0 1 2
31.	0 1 2 ?	0 1 2	**65.**	0 1 2 ?	0 1 2
32.	0 1 2 ? NA	0 1 2	**66.**	0 1 2 ?	0 1 2
33.	0 1 2 ? NA	0 1 2	**67.**	0 1 2 ?	0 1 2
34.	0 1 2 ?	0 1 2			

IPDE ICD-10 module handscoring algorithms and summary scoresheet

Directions

Transcribe the scores from the IPDE interview schedule or answer sheet to the scoresheet as follows:

1. Follow the item sequence on the scoresheet not the interview.
2. If there is a score based on informants *always* transcribe it instead of the score recorded during the interview. Identify an informant score on the scoresheets by placing it in [ ].
3. If you used the optional X and X̲ notation for recording past personality disorders, transcribe all such scores as 0 regardless of the actual score recorded on the interview schedule or answer sheet.
4. Enter scores of 0, ?, NA, and *circled* scores of 1 and 2 in the first column (<25), and *underlined* scores of 1 and 2 in the second column (≥ 25).
5. Begin by transcribing the scores for *F60.0 Paranoid*. Then follow the instructions on the scoresheets.

F60.0   Paranoid

Criteria		Items	Onset	
			<25	≥25
(1)	Excessive sensitivity to setbacks and rebuffs	38	_____	_____
(2)	Tendency to bear grudges persistently	34	_____	_____
(3)	Suspiciousness and tendency to distort	35	_____	_____
(4)	Combative, tenacious sense of personal rights	31	_____	_____
(5)	Suspiciousness regarding sexual fidelity	55	_____	_____
(6)	Self-important, self-referential attitude	36	_____	_____
(7)	Preoccupation with conspiratorial explanations	57	_____	_____

Diagnosis: Definite _____ Probable _____ Negative _____
Number of Criteria Met _____ **Dimensional Score** _____
Number of Criteria Based on Informant(s) _____

1. Count the number of scores in [ ], and enter the total after *Number of Criteria Based on Informant(s)*.
2. If there is no positive score (1 or 2) in column 1, enter 0 after *Number of Criteria Met* and *Dimensional Score*, check *Diagnosis Negative*, and go to next disorder, F60.1 Schizoid.
3. Add the scores in columns 1 and 2, and enter the sum after *Dimensional Score*.
4. If there is no score of 2 in column 1, enter 0 after *Number of Criteria Met*, check *Diagnosis Negative*, and go to next disorder, F60.1 Schizoid.
5. Count the number of 2s in columns 1 and 2, and enter the number after *Number of Criteria Met*.
6. If the number of criteria met is less than 3, check *Diagnosis Negative*, and go to next disorder, F60.1 Schizoid.
7. If the number of criteria met ≥ 4, check *Diagnosis Definite*, and go to next disorder, F60.1 Schizoid.
8. Check *Diagnosis Probable*, and go to next disorder, F60.1 Schizoid.

F60.1   Schizoid

Criteria	Items	Onset	
		<25	≥25
(1) Few, if any, activities provide pleasure	42	___	___
(2) Emotional coldness or flattened affectivity	67	___	___
(3) Limited capacity to express tender feelings and anger	*	___	___
(4) Appearance of indifference to praise or criticism	37	___	___
(5) Little interest in sexual experiences with another	53	___	___
(6) Constance choice of solitary activities	22	___	___
(7) Preoccupation with fantasy and introspection	18	___	___
(8) No desire for or possession of close friends	19	___	___
(9) Insensitivity to social norms and conventions	66	___	___

Diagnosis: Definite _____ Probable _____ Negative _____
Number of Criteria Met _____ **Dimensional Score** _____
Number of Criteria Based on Informant(s) _____

1. Count the number of scores in [ ], and enter the total after *Number of Criteria Based on Informant(s)*.
2. If there is no positive score (1 or 2) in column 1, enter 0 after *Number of Criteria Met* and *Dimensional Score*, check *Diagnosis Negative*, and go to next disorder, F60.2 Dissocial.
3. Add the scores in columns 1 and 2, and enter the sum after *Dimensional Score*.
4. If there is no score of 2 in column 1, enter 0 after *Number of Criteria Met*, check *Diagnosis Negative*, and go to next disorder, F60.2 Dissocial.
5. Count the number of 2s in columns 1 and 2, and enter the number after *Number of Criteria Met*.
6. If the number of criteria met is less than 3, check *Diagnosis Negative*, and go to next disorder, F60.2 Dissocial.
7. If the number of criteria met ≥ 4, check *Diagnosis Definite*, and go to next disorder, F60.2 Dissocial.
8. Check *Diagnosis Probable*, and go to next disorder, F60.1 Dissocial.

*   39+44=4,   score 2   39=1,44=0, score 0
    39+44=3,   score 2   39=0,44=1, score 0
    39=1,44=1, score 1   39=0,44=0, score 0

When combining the partial components of criterion (3), it is only necessary that one of the items occurs in the past 12 months and before age 25 years, for the score to be entered in the <25 column.

F60.2   Dissocial

Criteria	Items	Onset	
		<25	≥25
(1) Callous unconcern for feelings of others	29	_____	_____
(2) Irresponsibility and disregard for social norms	61	_____	_____
(3) Incapacity to maintain enduring relationships	20	_____	_____
(4) Low tolerance to frustration; aggressiveness	*	_____	_____
(5) No guilt and ability to profit from experience	**	_____	_____
(6) Marked proneness to rationalize behaviour	63	_____	_____

Diagnosis: Definite _____ Probable _____ Negative _____
Number of Criteria Met _____ **Dimensional Score** _____
Number of Criteria Based on Informant(s) _____

1. Count the number of scores in [ ], and enter the total after *Number of Criteria Based on Informant(s)*.
2. If there is no positive score (1 or 2) in column 1, enter 0 after *Number of Criteria Met* and *Dimensional Score*, check *Diagnosis Negative*, and go to next disorder, F60.30 Emotionally Unstable, Impulsive Type.
3. Add the scores in columns 1 and 2, and enter the sum after *Dimensional Score*.
4. If there is no score of 2 in column 1, enter 0 after *Number of Criteria Met*, check *Diagnosis Negative*, and go to next disorder, F60.30 Emotionally Unstable, Impulsive Type.
5. Count the number of 2s in columns 1 and 2, and enter the number after *Number of Criteria Met*.
6. If the number of criteria met is less than 2, check *Diagnosis Negative*, and go to next disorder, F60.30 Emotionally Unstable, Impulsive Type.
7. If the number of criteria met ≥ 3, check *Diagnosis Definite*, and go to next disorder, F60.30 Emotionally Unstable, Impulsive Type.
8. Check *Diagnosis Probable*, and go to next disorder, F60.30 Emotionally Unstable, Impulsive Type.

* 15+60=4, score 2	** 62+64=4, score 2
15+60=3, score 1	62+64=3, score 1
15+60=2, score 1	62+64=2, score 1
15+60=1, score 0	62+64=1, score 0
15+60=0, score 0	62+64=0, score 0

When combining the partial components of criteria (4) and (5), it is only necessary that one item occurs in the past 12 months and before age 25 years, for the score to be entered in the <25 column.

F60.30 **Emtionally Unstable, Impulsive Type**

Criteria	Items	Onset	
		<25	≥25
(1) Acts unexpectedly	58	___	___
(2) Quarrelsome when thwarted or criticized	30	___	___
(3) Liability to outbursts of anger or violence	43	___	___
(4) Not persistent when no immediate reward	11	___	___
(5) Unstable and capricious mood	50	___	___

Diagnosis: Definite _____ Probable _____ Negative _____
Number of Criteria Met _____ **Dimensional Score** _____
Number of Criteria Based on Informant(s) _____

1. Count the number of scores in [ ], and enter the total after *Number of Criteria Based on Informant(s)*.
2. If there is no positive score (1 or 2) in column 1, enter 0 after *Number of Criteria Met* and *Dimensional Score*, check *Diagnosis Negative*, and go to next disorder, F60.31 Emotionally Unstable, Borderline type.
3. Add the scores in columns 1 and 2, and enter the sum after *Dimensional Score*.
4. If there is no score of 2 in column 1, enter 0 after *Number of Criteria Met*, check *Diagnosis Negative*, and go to next disorder, F60.31 Emotionally Unstable, Borderline type.
5. Count the number of 2s in columns 1 and 2, and enter the number after *Number of Criteria Met*.
6. If item 30 is not scored 2, check *Diagnosis Negative*, and go to next disorder, F60.31 Emotionally Unstable, Borderline type.
7. If the number of criteria met is less than 2, check *Diagnosis Negative*, and go to next disorder, F60.31 Emotionally Unstable, Borderline Type.
8. If the number of criteria met ≥ 3, check *Diagnosis Definite*, and go to next disorder, F60.31 Emotionally Unstable, Borderline type.
9. Check *Diagnosis Probable*, and go to next disorder, F60.31 Emotionally Unstable, Borderline type.

F60.31   Emotionally Unstable, Borderline Type

Criteria	Items	Onset <25	Onset ≥25
(1) Acts unexpectedly	58	_____	_____
(2) Quarrelsome when thwarted or criticized	30	_____	_____
(3) Liability to anger or violence	43	_____	_____
(4) Not persistent when no immediate reward	11	_____	_____
(5) Unstable and capricious mood	50	_____	_____
(6) Uncertainty about self-image, aims, etc	*	_____	_____
(7) Intense and unstable relationships	26	_____	_____
(8) Excessive efforts to avoid abandonment	48	_____	_____
(9) Recurrent threats or acts of self-harm	59	_____	_____
(10) Chronic feelings of emptiness	45	_____	_____

Diagnosis: Definite _____ Probable _____ Negative _____
Number of Criteria Met _____ **Dimensional Score** _____
Number of Criteria Based on Informant(s) _____

1. Count the number of scores in [ ], and enter the total after *Number of Criteria Based on Informant(s)*.
2. If there is no positive score (1 or 2) in column 1, enter 0 after *Number of Criteria Met* and *Dimensional Score*, check *Diagnosis Negative*, and go to next disorder, F60.4 Histrionic.
3. Add the scores in columns 1 and 2, and enter the sum after *Dimensional Score*.
4. If there is no score of 2 in column 1, enter 0 after *Number of Criteria Met*, check *Diagnosis Negative*, and go to next disorder, F60.4 Histrionic.
5. Count the number of 2s in columns 1 and 2, and enter the number after *Number of Criteria Met*.
6. If the number of criteria 1-5 met ≥ 3 and the number of criteria 6-10 met ≥ 2, check *Diagnosis Definite*, and go to next disorder, F60.4 Histrionic.
7. If the number of criteria 1-5 met is less than 2 and the number of criteria 6-10 met is less than 2, check *Diagnosis Negative*, and go to next disorder, F60.4 Histrionic.
8. Check *Diagnosis Probable*, and go to next disorder, F60.4 Histrionic.

* 5, 6, 7, 25, 56
two or more scores of 2, score 2
one score of 2, score 1
no scores of 2, but sum ≥ 3, score 1
all others, score 0

When combining the partial components of criterion 6, it is only necessary that one item occurs in the past 12 months and before age 25 years, for the score to be entered in the <25 column.

F60.4   Histrionic

Criteria	Items	Onset	
		<25	≥25
(1) Self-dramatization, exaggerated emotional display	40	_____	_____
(2) Suggestibility, easily influenced	12	_____	_____
(3) Shallow and labile affectivity	49	_____	_____
(4) Seeks excitement and attention	*	_____	_____
(5) Inappropriate seductiveness in appearance or behaviour	54	_____	_____
(6) Over concern with physical attractiveness	17	_____	_____

Diagnosis: Definite _____ Probable _____ Negative _____
Number of Criteria Met _____ **Dimensional Score** _____
Number of Criteria Based on Informant(s) _____

1.   Count the number of scores in [ ], and enter the total after *Number of Criteria Based on Informant(s)*.
2.   If there is no positive score (1 or 2) in column 1, enter 0 after *Number of Criteria Met* and *Dimensional Score*, check *Diagnosis Negative*, and go to next disorder, F60.5 Anankastic.
3.   Add the scores in columns 1 and 2, and enter the sum after *Dimensional Score*.
4.   If there is no score of 2 in column 1, enter 0 after *Number of Criteria Met*, check *Diagnosis Negative*, and go to next disorder, F60.5 Anankastic.
5.   Count the number of 2s in columns 1 and 2, and enter the number after *Number of Criteria Met*.
6.   If the number of criteria met is less than 3, check *Diagnosis Negative*, and go to next disorder, F60.5 Anankastic.
7.   If the number of criteria met ≥ 4, check *Diagnosis Definite*, and go to next disorder, F60.5 Anankastic.
8.   Check *Diagnosis Probable*, and go to next disorder, F60.5 Anankastic.

*   16+41=4, score 2
      16+41=3, score 1
      16+41=2, score 1
      16+41=1, score 0
      16+41=0, score 0

When combining the partial components of criterion (4), it is only necessary that one item occurs in the past 12 months and before age 25 years, for the score to be entered in the <25 column.

F60.5   Anankastic

Criteria	Items	Onset <25	Onset ≥25
(1) Excessive doubt and caution	9	_____	_____
(2) Preoccupation with detail	3	_____	_____
(3) Perfectionism	2	_____	_____
(4) Excessive conscientiousness and scrupulousness	14	_____	_____
(5) Undue preoccupation with productivity	1	_____	_____
(6) Pedantry and conventionality	65	_____	_____
(7) Rigidity and stubbornness	28	_____	_____
(8) Insistence on doing things own way	27	_____	_____

Diagnosis: Definite _____ Probable _____ Negative _____
Number of Criteria Met _____ **Dimensional Score** _____
Number of Criteria Based on Informant(s) _____

1. Count the number of scores in [ ], and enter the total after *Number of Criteria Based on Informant(s)*.
2. If there is no positive score (1 or 2) in column 1, enter 0 after *Number of Criteria Met* and *Dimensional Score*, check *Diagnosis Negative*, and go to next disorder, F60.6 Anxious.
3. Add the scores in columns 1 and 2, and enter the sum after *Dimensional Score*.
4. If there is no score of 2 in column 1, enter 0 after *Number of Criteria Met*, check *Diagnosis Negative*, and go to next disorder, F60.6 Anxious.
5. Count the number of 2s in columns 1 and 2, and enter the number after *Number of Criteria Met*.
6. If the number of criteria met is less than 3, check *Diagnosis Negative*, and go to next disorder, F60.6 Anxious.
7. If the number of criteria met ≥ 4, check *Diagnosis Definite*, and go to next disorder, F60.6 Anxious.
8. Check *Diagnosis Probable*, and go to next disorder, F60.6 Anxious.

F60.6   Anxious [avoidant]

Criteria		Items	Onset	
			<25	≥25
(1)	Persistent, pervasive feelings of tension	52	_____	_____
(2)	Feels socially inept and inferior	13	_____	_____
(3)	Preoccupied with criticism or rejection	24	_____	_____
(4)	Social avoidance if doesn't feel liked	23	_____	_____
(5)	Need for security restricts lifestyle	51	_____	_____
(6)	Social avoidance due to fear of rejection	*	_____	_____

Diagnosis: Definite _____ Probable _____ Negative _____
Number of Criteria Met _____ **Dimensional Score** _____
Number of Criteria Based on Informant(s) _____

1. Count the number of scores in [ ], and enter the total after *Number of Criteria Based on Informant(s)*.
2. If there is no positive score (1 or 2) in column 1, enter 0 after *Number of Criteria Met* and *Dimensional Score*, check *Diagnosis Negative*, and go to next disorder, F60.7 Dependent.
3. Add the scores in columns 1 and 2, and enter the sum after *Dimensional Score*.
4. If there is no score of 2 in column 1, enter 0 after *Number of Criteria Met*, check *Diagnosis Negative*, and go to next disorder, F60.7 Dependent.
5. Count the number of 2s in columns 1 and 2, and enter the number after *Number of Criteria Met*.
6. If the number of criteria met is less than 3, check *Diagnosis Negative*, and go to next disorder, F60.7 Dependent.
7. If the number of criteria met ≥ 4, check *Diagnosis Definite*, and go to next disorder, F60.7 Dependent.
8. Check *Diagnosis Probable*, and go to next disorder, F60.7 Dependent.

*   4+21=4, score 2
      4+21=3, score 1
      4+21=2, score 1
      4+21=1, score 0
      4+21=0, score 0

When combining the partial components of criterion (6), it is only necessary that one item occurs in the past 12 months and before age 25 years, for the score to be entered in the <25 column.

F60.7   Dependent

Criteria	Items	Onset	
		<25	≥25
(1) Allowing others to make one's important decisions	10	___	___
(2) Subordinates own needs to those on whom dependent	33	___	___
(3) Unwilling to demand from those on whom dependent	32	___	___
(4) Uncomfortable or helpless when alone	46	___	___
(5) Fears abandonment	47	___	___
(6) Needs excessive advice and reassurance	8	___	___

Diagnosis: Definite _____ Probable _____ Negative _____
Number of Criteria Met _____ **Dimensional Score** _____
Number of Criteria Based on Informant(s) _____

1. Count the number of scores in [ ], and enter the total after *Number of Criteria Based on Informant(s)*.
2. If there is no positive score (1 or 2) in column 1, enter 0 after *Number of Criteria Met* and *Dimensional Score*, check *Diagnosis Negative*, and to go next disorder, F60.9 Personality Disorder, Unspecified.
3. Add the scores in columns 1 and 2, and enter the sum after *Dimensional Score*.
4. If there is no score of 2 in column 1, enter 0 after *Number of Criteria Met*, check *Diagnosis Negative*, and go to next disorder, F60.9 Personality Disorder, Unspecified.
5. Count the number of 2s in columns 1 and 2, and enter the number after *Number of Criteria Met*.
6. If the number of criteria met is less than 3, check *Diagnosis Negative*, and go to next disorder, F60.9 Personality Disorder, Unspecified.
7. If the number of criteria met ≥ 4, check *Diagnosis Definite*, and either fill out the Summary Scoresheet, or go to the optional diagnoses.
8. Check *Diagnosis Probable*, and go to next disorder, F60.9 Personality Disorder, Unspecified.

F60.9   Personality Disorder, Unspecified

Diagnosis: Definite _____ Probable _____ Negative _____
Number of Criteria Met _____ **Dimensional Score** _____
Number of Criteria Based on Informant(s) _____

1. If there is a *Definite Diagnosis* for any specific personality disorder, check *Diagnosis Negative*, and either fill out the Summary Scoresheet, or go to the optional diagnoses.
2. Add the number of scores entered after *Number of Criteria Based on Informant(s)* on the scoresheets for the specific disorders, excluding Impulsive disorder, and enter the total after *Number of Criteria Based on Informant(s)*.
3. Add the number of criteria entered after *Number of Criteria Met* on the scoresheets for the specific disorders, excluding Impulsive disorder, and enter the total after *Number of Criteria Met*.
4. If the number of criteria met is less than 9, check *Diagnosis Negative*, and either fill out the Summary Scoresheet, or go to the optional diagnoses.
5. If the number of criteria met ≥ 10, check *Diagnosis Definite*, and either fill out the Summary Scoresheet, or go to the optional diagnoses.
6. Check *Diagnosis Probable*, and either fill out the Summary Scoresheet, or go to optional diagnoses.

Optional

Past Personality Disorders

Follow these steps with *each* disorder (except Emotionally Unstable and Unspecified) with no current *Definite* diagnosis:

1. Transcribe all the 2 scores recorded on the interview schedule or answer sheet with the X or X̲ notation, by placing an X or X̲ through the corresponding number in the Items column of the scoresheet for the disorder. Do *not* enter the scores in either column 1 (onset <25) or column 2 (onset ≥25).
2. If there are no 2 scores with an X or X̲ notation, enter 0 in Table 1 under *Number Criteria Met*, and go to next disorder.
3. If the number recorded next to *Number of Criteria Met* on the scoresheet is 0, and there is no 2 score with an X (not X̲) notation, enter 0 in Table 1 under *Number Criteria Met*, and go to next disorder.
4. Count the number of 2 scores with an X or X̲ in the Items column of the scoresheet, add the number recorded next to *Number of Criteria Met* on the scoresheet, and enter the sum in Table 1 under *Number Criteria Met*.
5. If the sum is ≥ than the number in parenthesis, check *Diagnosis Definite*, and go to next disorder.
6. If the sum is one less than the number in parenthesis, check *Diagnosis Probable*.
7. Go to next disorder.

Past Emotionally Unstable Disorder, Impulsive Type

1. If there is a current *Definite* diagnosis of Impulsive, go to Past Borderline disorder.
2. Transcribe all the 2 scores recorded on the interview schedule or answer sheet with the X or X̲ notation by placing an X or X̲ through the corresponding number in the Items column of the Impulsive scoresheet. Do *not* enter the scores in either column 1 (onset <25) or column 2 (onset ≥25).
3. If there are no Impulsive 2 scores with an X or X̲ notation, enter 0 in Table 1 under *Number Criteria Met*, and go to Past Borderline disorder.
4. If the number recorded next to *Number of Criteria Met* on the Impulsive scoresheet is 0, and there is no Impulsive 2 score with an X (not X̲) notation, enter 0 in Table 1 under *Number Criteria Met*, and go to Past Borderline disorder.
5. Count the number of 2 scores with an X or X̲ in the Items column of the Impulsive scoresheet, add the number recorded next to *Number of Criteria Met* on the scoresheet, and enter the sum in Table 1 under *Number Criteria Met*.
6. If the sum is less than 2, go to Past Borderline disorder.
7. If item 30 is not scored 2 *and* has no X or X̲ notation in the items column, go to Past Borderline disorder.
8. If the number of criteria met ≥ 3, check *Diagnosis Definite*, and go to Past Borderline disorder.
9. Check *Diagnosis Probable* and go to Past Borderline disorder.

Past Emotionally Unstable Disorder, Borderline Type

1. If there is a current *Definite* diagnosis of Borderline, either fill out the Summary Scoresheet, or go to Late Onset disorders.
2. Transcribe all the 2 scores recorded on the interview schedule or answer sheet with the X or X̲ notation by placing an X or X̲ through the corresponding number in the Items column of the Borderline scoresheet. Do *not* enter the scores in either column 1 (onset <25) or column 2 (onset ≥25).
3. If there are no Borderline 2 scores with an X or X̲ notation, enter 0 in Table 1 under *Number Criteria Met*, and go to Past Unspecified disorder.
4. If the number recorded next to *Number of Criteria Met* on the Borderline scoresheet is 0, and there is no Borderline 2 score with an X (not X̲) notation, enter 0 in Table 1 under *Number Criteria Met*, and go to Past Unspecified disorder.
5. Count the number of 2 scores with an X or X̲ notation in the Items column of the Borderline scoresheet, add the number recorded next to *Number of Criteria Met* on the scoresheet, and enter the sum in Table 1 under *Number Criteria Met*.
6. If the number of criteria 1-5 met is less than 2 and the number of criteria 6-10 met is less than 2, go to Past Unspecified disorder.
7. If the number of criteria 1-5 met ≥3 and the number of criteria 6-10 met ≥2, check *Diagnosis Definite*, and either fill out the Summary Scoresheet or go to Late Onset disorders.
8. Check *Diagnosis Probable*, and go to Past Unspecified disorder.

Past Unspecified Disorder

1. If there is a *Definite* diagnosis (current or past) for *any* personality disorder, either fill out the Summary Scoresheet or go to Late Onset disorders.
2. Add the numbers in Table 1 under *Number Criteria Met*, excluding Impulsive disorder, and enter the sum next to Unspecified.
3. If the sum is less than 9, either fill out the Summary Scoresheet or go to Late Onset disorders.
4. If the sum ≥10, check *Diagnosis Definite*, and either fill out the Summary Scoresheet or go to Late Onset disorders.
5. Check *Diagnosis Probable*, and either fill out the Summary Scoresheet or go to Late Onset disorders.

Table 1

	Number Criteria Met	Diagnosis Definite	Diagnosis Probable
F60.0 Paranoid ....(4)	_____	_____	_____
F60.1 Schizoid ....(4)	_____	_____	_____
F60.2 Dissocial........(3)	_____	_____	_____
F60.30 Emotionally Unstable, Impulsive type	_____	_____	_____
F60.31 Emotionally Unstable, Borderline type.....	_____	_____	_____
F60.4 Histrionic ......(4)	_____	_____	_____
F60.5 Anankastic....(4)	_____	_____	_____
F60.6 Anxious..........(4)	_____	_____	_____
F60.7 Dependent ...(4)	_____	_____	_____
F60.9 Unspecified	_____	_____	_____

Optional

Late Onset Personality Disorders

Follow these steps with *each* disorder (except Emotionally Unstable and Unspecified) with no *Definite* diagnosis (current or past) *and* no score of 2 in column 1 (onset<25) of the scoresheet for the disorder:

1. Count the number of 2 scores in column 2 (onset ≥25) of the scoresheet, and enter the number in Table 2 under *Number Criteria Met*.
2. If the number of criteria met > the number in parenthesis, check *Diagnosis Definite*, and go to next disorder.
3. If the number of criteria met is one less than the number in parenthesis, check *Diagnosis Probable*.
4. Go to next disorder.

Late Onset Emotionally Unstable Disorder, Impulsive Type

1. If there is a *Definite* diagnosis (current or past) of Impulsive, go to Late Onset Borderline disorder.
2. If there is a score of 2 in column 1 (onset <25) of the Impulsive scoresheet, go to Late Onset Borderline disorder.
3. If there is no score of 2 in column 2 (onset ≥25) of the Impulsive scoresheet, go to Late Onset Borderline disorder.
4. Count the number of 2 scores in column 2 (onset ≥25) of the Impulsive scoresheet, and enter the number in Table 2 under *Number Criteria Met*.
5. If item 30 is not scored 2 in either onset column (<25 or ≥25), go to Late Onset Borderline disorder.
6. If the number of criteria met is less than 2, go to Late Onset Borderline disorder.
7. If the number of criteria met ≥3, check *Diagnosis Definite*, and go to Late Onset Borderline disorder.
8. Check *Diagnosis Probable*, and go to Late Onset Borderline disorder.

Late Onset Emotionally Unstable Disorder, Borderline Type

1. If there is a *Definite* diagnosis (current or past) of Borderline, go to Late Onset Unspecified disorder.
2. If there is a score of 2 in column 1 (onset <25) of the Borderline scoresheet, go to Late Onset Unspecified disorder.
3. If there is no score of 2 in column 2 (onset ≥25) of the Borderline scoresheet, go to Late Onset Unspecified disorder.
4. Count the number of 2 scores in column 2 (onset ≥25) of the Borderline scoresheet, and enter the number in Table 2 under *Number Criteria Met*.
5. If the number of criteria 1-5 met is less than 2 and the number of criteria 6-10 met is less than 2, go to Late Onset Unspecified disorder.
6. If the number of criteria 1-5 met ≥3 and the number of criteria 6-10 met ≥2, check *Diagnosis Definite*, and fill out the Summary Scoresheet.
7. Check *Diagnosis Probable*, and go to Late Onset Unspecified Disorder.

Late Onset Personality Disorder, Unspecified

1. If there is a *Definite Diagnosis* for any specific personality disorder (current or past), check *Diagnosis Negative*, and fill out the Summary Scoresheet.
2. Add the number of scores entered after *Number of Criteria Based on Informant(s)* on the scoresheets for the specific disorders, excluding Impulsive disorder, and enter the total after *Number of Criteria Based on Informant(s)*.
3. Add the number of criteria entered after *Number of Criteria Met* on the scoresheets for the specific disorders, excluding Impulsive disorder, and enter the total after *Number of Criteria Met*.
4. If the number of criteria met is less than 9, check *Diagnosis Negative*, and fill out the Summary Scoresheet.
5. If the number of criteria met ≥10, check *Diagnosis Definite*, and fill out the Summary Scoresheet.
6. Check *Diagnosis Probable*, and fill out the Summary Scoresheet.

Table 2

		Number Criteria Met	Diagnosis Definite	Diagnosis Probable
F60.0	Paranoid ....(4)	_____	_____	_____
F60.1	Schizoid ....(4)	_____	_____	_____
F60.2	Dissocial........(3)	_____	_____	_____
F60.30	Emotionally Unstable, Impulsive type	_____	_____	_____
F60.31	Emotionally Unstable, Borderline type.....	_____	_____	_____
F60.4	Histrionic ......(4)	_____	_____	_____
F60.5	Anankastic....(4)	_____	_____	_____
F60.6	Anxious.........(4)	_____	_____	_____
F60.7	Dependent ...(4)	_____	_____	_____
F60.9	Unspecified	_____	_____	_____

IPDE ICD-10 module summary scoresheet

Last Name   First Name   Middle Initial

Sex: _____   Age: _____   Marital Status: _____

Education: _____   Occupation: _____

Examiner   Date(s)   Time Required for Interview

		Summary	Diagnosis			
ICD-10 Disorder	Number Criteria Met	Dimensional Score	Definite	Probable	Negative	Confidence Rating
F60.0 Paranoid	_____	_____	_____	_____	_____	_____
F60.1 Schizoid	_____	_____	_____	_____	_____	_____
F60.2 Dissocial	_____	_____	_____	_____	_____	_____
F60.30 Emotionally unstable Impulsive type	_____	_____	_____	_____	_____	_____
F60.31 Emotionally unstable Borderline type	_____	_____	_____	_____	_____	_____
F60.4 Histrionic	_____	_____	_____	_____	_____	_____
F60.5 Anankastic	_____	_____	_____	_____	_____	_____
F60.6 Anxious	_____	_____	_____	_____	_____	_____
F60.7 Dependent	_____	_____	_____	_____	_____	_____
F60.9 Unspecified	_____	_____	_____	_____	_____	_____

For each disorder check one: **Definite**, **Probable**, or **Negative**. If using the optional scoring, indicate next to the check mark, when a *Definite* or *Probable* diagnosis is **past**, **late onset**, or **past late onset**.

Rate your level of confidence (1=High, 2=Moderate, 3=Low) in the validity of every diagnostic decision, using your clinical judgment, the IPDE interview, and other information when available.

Index